The Project 2000 Nurse
The Remaking of British General Nursing 1978–2000

T0385535

The Project 2000 Nurse

The Remaking of British General Nursing 1978–2000

ANN BRADSHAW PhD, SRN, DipN(Lond)

Oxford Brookes University

W

WHURR PUBLISHERS

LONDON AND PHILADELPHIA

© 2001 Whurr Publishers
First published 2001 by
Whurr Publishers Ltd
19в Compton Terrace, London N1 2UN, England and
325 Chestnut Street, Philadelphia PA 19106, USA

British Library Cataloguing in Publication Data
A catalogue record for this book is available from the
British Library.

ISBN 978-1-86156-222-7

FSC
Mixed Sources
Product group from well-managed
forests and other controlled sources
Cert no. SGS-COC-2953
www.fsc.org
© 1996 Forest Stewardship Council

Contents

Foreword   vii
Lord Morris of Castle Morris

Introduction   xi

Chapter 1   1

The background and context for change – the end of the
apprenticeship tradition

Chapter 2   18

The autonomous practitioner – statutory and educational changes
1981–1986

Chapter 3   47

Educating for competence? Nurse education 1985–1999

Chapter 4   85

'Professionhood', vocation and new nursing roles 1990–1999

Chapter 5   114

Shortage of nurses and concerns over the quality of patient care
1994–1999

Chapter 6   **151**

Parliamentary reaction to Project 2000 and the nursing system
1990–2000

Conclusion   **185**

The paradox of nursing at the year 2000

References   **193**
Index   **223**

Foreword

At 7.59 p.m., 16 June 1998, the Clerk of the Parliaments announced the next debate on the House of Lords Order Paper, on 'Nurses in the NHS', which I was to open. 'The Lord Morris of Castle Morris,' he called in ringing tones. I rose, and caused a minor sensation by saying, 'Not so, my Lords. I am not what I seem. I am Number 445590, Morris, Brian, d.o.b. 04:12:30, male, C of E. I know this because it was written on the little plastic bracelet placed on my wrist on 21 January last, when I became a patient in the Royal Hospital, Chesterfield, whence I came this morning to ask the question standing in my name.' Well, it was a way of getting their Lordships' attention, and I wanted to make the point that in an NHS hospital all persons are equal, and there is neither Greek nor Jew, Barbarian, Scythian, bond nor free.

It was an important little debate. Many of the heavyweights of the nursing profession contributed, including Baroness McFarlane, Baroness Emerton, Baroness Masham, Lord Hunt, Earl Howe, and Baroness Jay. It was part of a campaign to get more money *for* (and directly *to*) the nurses in the NHS. And, sure enough, thanks to the coincidence of a campaign on the same subject by the indefatigable journalists of the *Daily Mail*, the Government awarded all nurses a pay rise of 3.8 per cent and some got even more.

That debate, and one or two others I was able to contribute to, were read by Dr Ann Bradshaw, author of this excellent and timely book, who has paid me the great compliment of asking me to write a foreword to it. She sent me the typescript, and I read every word of it, realizing – as a former university Professor of English – that I had before me a scholarly work of high quality, which had the additional advantage of being clearly and elegantly written.

Dr Bradshaw chronicles in detail the attempt, over the past quarter century, to 'professionalize' nursing. From Florence Nightingale to the 1960s, nurses were recruited and trained on what can be loosely described as the 'apprenticeship' system. Most of their training took place in hospitals and on the ward, most of their teachers were doctors or nurses. During the 1960s, for a variety of reasons, nurses (and especially the leaders of nurses) became ambitious to secure recognition and increased status for their work. Nursing was becoming steadily more and more technical, academic and responsible, and accountable. This laudable desire was recognized and approved by the sensitive antennae of politicians of all parties. The watershed was the Briggs Report of 1972, which decisively dismantled the apprenticeship system, broke up the previous common syllabus, allowed universities and other training bodies to develop their own curricula, and aimed to produce nurses as 'students', like students on university liberal arts courses. They were to become independent, autonomous, self-motivated, self-developing, creative, flexible and self-critical. Their studies were to include psychology, sociology, educational philosophy, and examinations were to be totally different from the tests of the past. Nurse education (it was prophesied) would become more theoretical, more academic, without sacrificing any of the practical skills necessary for patient care. As an RCN report put it, students should no longer be overworked 'pairs of hands' whose own learning needs were secondary because they marched 'to the drumbeat of service'.

For the next quarter of a century this new approach to nursing – as a secular profession, not a vocation – was developed, varied, experimented with, and endlessly discussed. Research papers, articles in the nursing press, reports from the Royal College of Nursing (RCN), the English National Board for Nursing, Midwifery and Health Visiting (ENB) and the United Kingdom Central Council for Nursing, Midwifery and Health Visiting (UKCC) thudded on to desks, negotiating tables and into libraries to be anaesthetised, operated on, placed in intensive care and monitored hourly. The pros and cons were disputed minutely and endlessly. Dr Bradshaw lists them comprehensively and describes them patiently, clearly and disinterestedly. In this she makes a major contribution to the history of nursing and her book is sure to become the standard reference work on the subject.

The conclusions she draws, in the later chapters, are the result of this careful analysis. Fundamentally, she argues, 'the reliance on the nurse's moral character, "a good nurse being a good woman", was no longer seen as relevant to nurse preparation. Contract had replaced covenant . . .' But, and this is the heart of the matter, *the contractual model has been unable to sustain the ethic of compassionate care'*. Compassion is an inconvenient concept: it cannot be measured, rationed or costed. It cannot be planned or delivered, but it will not go away.

I had reason to be regularly reminded of this when I spent two periods of about five months each as a patient in an NHS hospital. Only a few days after I was admitted we were all distressed and sleepless because a young man with severe head injuries kept up a nerve-racking unearthly wailing noise for hours on end, and no form of sedation seemed to help. In the end, a nurse came in, sat on his bed, put both arms around him and cuddled him for an hour. She rocked him gently, like a baby, and murmured things to him. His mind was too far away to know what was happening, but the simple human contact, the compassion, calmed him and relieved him when no drug had been effective.

You cannot teach compassion. In nurse education there is no instruction in 'tender, loving care'. The post-Briggs developments begat Project 2000, which was acutely aware of the need for a solid academic element in nurse education. To psychology and sociology was added competence in the fast-developing new technology, but in its drive for a new concept of 'autonomous professional competence' nurse education failed to create and win acceptance for a new 'image' to which the nurse could relate or aspire. There may have been, in the minds of the educators, some fuzzy picture of the calm, self-confident, poised young woman, deploying at the bedside her achieved sociological skills and technological expertise with complicated machinery, diagnosing and prescribing for her patients, and advising her consultants as to alternative regimes of treatment. But this icon has not won and never will win acceptance, because it simply does not reflect the daily realities of life on the ward.

The concept of a nurse's 'status' must be considered far more profoundly, imaginatively and (dare I say it) *poetically* than it has been over the past 20 years. I offer one, perhaps rather strange, example from my own hospital experience. We had a middle-aged, experienced staff nurse, who was 'acting up' as sister in charge of the ward for the afternoon shift. It was understaffed and work was hectic. Her young nurses were flying about dealing with a series of emergencies. In the midst of this I suddenly caught sight of her walking slowly and calmly down the ward to the sluice room carrying before her a bedpan covered with a length of toilet paper. Nothing special in that, but the image stayed in my mind. A few days later I saw the hospital chaplain on his rounds, taking communion to the patients, carrying before him the paten and chalice, covered with the burse and veil. The contrast between faeces and sacrament could not have been greater: the comparison of the two 'icons of service' could hardly have been more striking. Ever since Florence Nightingale, the 'lady of the lamp', there have been images of the nurse, usually of the 'angel of mercy' type, but these have become outmoded. I would not want to suggest that a new iconography should prominently feature the bedpan, but there is a crying need for some new picture epitomizing the essence of what a nurse is and does.

The most powerful element in the backlash against the post-Briggs model for nursing work came, however, in the reaction against the concept of the 'autonomous' nurse. Granted that specialist nurses (district nurses, health visitors and the like) spend much of their time working alone and must be held responsible for their decisions, the great majority of nurses work in hospitals, and in teams. Before 1972, there was a clear structure of authority: SEN, SRN, Staff Nurse, Sister, Matron. Sister was in charge of the ward, and Matron was in charge of all nurses and nursing. In sundry ways and for various reasons this hierarchy has been steadily dismantled over the past nearly 30 years, and this has led to growing unease – especially since the rise of litigation against hospital staff.

Perhaps the fault lies in the insistence upon professionalization, when there is no clear sense of what a profession is. *The Oxford English Dictionary* (s.v. Profession, III, 6a) states:

> A vocation in which a professed knowledge of some department of learning or science is used in application to the affairs of others or in the practice of an art founded upon it. Applied spec. to the three learned professions of divinity, law, and medicine; also to the military profession.

This confounds the confusion, first by describing a profession as a vocation (nursing as a 'vocation' has been a concept fiercely resisted in the period since 1972) and second by asserting the 'profession' of medicine (of which, presumably, nursing is essentially a sub-set). Until these questions of status and hierarchy are resolved there can be no clear understanding of the nurse's role.

Most Parliamentarians read the Parliamentary weekly, *The House Magazine*. The issue for 19 June 2000 is devoted to health care, and features an article by Lord McColl of Dulwich, CBE, a Conservative peer and front bench spokesman on the NHS. It begins:

> If I were in charge of the NHS, I would be trying to bring back matron, or matron's values. I would insist that hospitals were cleaned . . . And I would try to emphasise the idea that the patient is the centre of the medical universe.

Although he and I might disagree on many things I would accept every word of that. And I suspect that Dr Ann Bradshaw, who has thought so long and deeply about the subject, might agree with us both.

Morris
House of Lords
January 2001

Introduction

On 1 November 1978 the Queen addressed Parliament. Her speech announced the government's intention to introduce a Bill on the regulation and training of the nursing, midwifery and health visiting professions, on the lines recommended by the Briggs Committee on nursing (House of Lords, Queen's Speech, 1978: 8). This date marks the point of formal ending of the past apprenticeship tradition of nursing. The last syllabus of the General Nursing Council was issued in 1977, and the following year saw the point of inception of the new system of nursing, with which this book deals.

The new regulatory structure which replaced the General Nursing Council, the United Kingdom Central Council for Nursing, Midwifery and Health Visiting (UKCC), bore fruit in the form of a radical new system of British nurse education introduced from 1986, and entitled Project 2000. Project 2000 was a root and branch replacement of the apprenticeship tradition of nurse training and its defining values, which began at St Thomas's Hospital in 1860, formed the nursing system in the UK for a century, and which has had a worldwide impact and influence. Project 2000 fulfilled its name on 1 January 2000, a significant and appropriate moment, therefore, to review its effectiveness.

By 1999 intense debates on British nursing and nurse education were occurring at both governmental and professional levels. A 'new model' of nurse education was to commence in September 2000, a new regulatory body for nursing was to be in place by 2001, and a major revision of the nursing role and its possible replacement was being suggested by academic thinkers. At the same time, serious concerns were being voiced about the quality of some nursing care. As the year 2000 arrived, there were many unanswered questions about the shape, ethos and future direction of the British nursing profession.

This book sets the historical, ethical, cultural and political contexts for the debate and develops a coherent analysis of the period of fundamental change in the nursing profession between 1978 and 2000. Parliamentary debates, professional and governmental reports, documents and studies, as well as opinions expressed in nursing and medical journals, illuminate this period of nursing. The review sets out to be both comprehensive and systematic, and there are no intentional omissions. Comment is kept to a minimum in order to allow the evidence to speak for itself and so enable the reader to make his or her own judgement on the evidence presented. Not only does this analysis have relevance for modern British nursing, but because of the British influence on nursing worldwide, it has contemporary international significance. In order to reach the depth necessary for systematic analysis, where this becomes necessary, England is taken as a representative example of the nationwide effects of the changes to nursing.

Chapter 1 sets out the model of nurse training that preceded the current system. It discusses the values and practices of the apprenticeship tradition, with particular regard to traditional vocational values. The system of training nurses for this purpose involved four principles: the development of moral character; the building up of technical knowledge, practical skill, routine and procedure; the authority, influence and supervision of the ward sister; and the induction into the professional etiquette of right relationships. Criticisms of this approach in the 1960s and 1970s formed a powerful critique which challenged the old system, and led to the introduction of what was perceived to be a more professional approach.

Chapter 2 examines the new nursing values that were introduced in the early 1980s and gave rise to Project 2000 and the supernumerary nurse. These values were the basis for key proposals from the Royal College of Nursing, the English National Board for Nursing, Midwifery and Health Visiting, and the UKCC, and formed the new policy for nursing preparation. The political response is analysed, particularly with regard to provisos made by government. The medical profession and grass-roots nurses were disturbed by the proposals; their concerns are charted and analysed.

Chapter 3 considers modern nursing education and preparation for competence since the introduction of Project 2000. Nursing leaders had sought a new structure for education befitting new forms of self-regulation. The individual learner was to take responsibility for his or her own learning. Optimistically it was thought the nursing student would be self-motivated, self-developing, creative, flexible and self-critical; but this optimism proved to be questionable. Evidence shows that the competence needed by the registered nurse was not defined by the new system. As a result there were serious concerns about whether nurse education prepared nurses to be fit to practise. One significant consequence of the new system of education is revealed to be the way in which it has undermined the role of the ward sister.

Chapter 4 investigates 'professionhood', vocation and new nursing roles. Changes in nurse preparation have been accompanied by a blurring of nursing roles. Health care assistants have increasingly taken on duties that traditionally had belonged to nurses, while nurses have taken on tasks that were previously performed by doctors. Proposals for a future health care workforce have sought to break down barriers between professions, with further questions over preparation for competence. The consequence has been confusion and fragmentation in the nursing role. Despite these status-driven changes, evidence has continued to show that many nurses maintain a deeply ingrained concept of vocation. The new system of nurse preparation held within it four key contradictions, as the discussion demonstrates.

Chapter 5 examines the issues of nursing shortages and quality in care. An important justification for the introduction of Project 2000 was the argument that increased status would improve recruitment and retention, even though it was admitted that this was not a problem at the time. As a consequence it was believed that patient care would benefit. This chapter examines these two issues, a decade after the implementation of Project 2000. Evidence reveals serious nursing shortages and crises in recruitment and retention over the following decade. There is also mounting evidence of inadequate nursing care, particularly of the elderly and vulnerable. An important issue for discussion is the extent to which shortcomings may be attributable to the loss of the vocational ethos in nursing, in turn reflecting the changed values in society. The ethos of vocation, once regarded as emphasizing the status of the person needing to be cared for in sanctifying and consecrating the caring act, is contrasted with the professionalized market-based approach to nursing, and the commodification of caring. This raises important questions about the nature and underpinning values of nursing as personal care for sick and vulnerable people.

Chapter 6 explores the parliamentary response to nursing changes through the 1990s. In 1979 the government had devolved responsibility to the profession for its own self-regulation. By the 1990s parliamentary debate showed a gradual concern about nursing developments, and weaknesses in self-regulation, and by 1997 these concerns brought about a review of the nursing legislation. Evidence from parliamentary debates and government publications shows ambivalence and a lack of clarity about the nature, purpose and direction of nursing in addressing and meeting public need. This is revealed to be the key issue confronting the nursing profession in the twenty-first century.

The conclusion draws together the preceding analysis to raise questions about the direction of nursing, the role of the nurse, and the method for preparation. This summation relates the analysis to the previous model of training, drawing comparisons in four areas: the nature of education, the role of the ward sister, professional relationships, and the place of vocation. It emerges from this that nursing at the start of year 2000 was confronted by five paradoxes, regarding recruitment and retention; education; regulation; professionalization and vocation; and the centrality of patient care. This analysis forms a basis for reflection on the future of the nursing profession.

For the sake of convenience, and where necessary, the female gender will be used to refer to the nurse; this convention should be taken as including male nurses who constitute a minority.

CHAPTER 1

The background and context for change – the end of the apprenticeship tradition

Introduction

British nurse training was an apprenticeship system, controlled through statutory syllabuses and informed by nursing textbooks. The syllabuses demonstrated the formal curriculum, specified by the statutory body of nursing, the General Nursing Council. This was mandatory in all nurse training schools in England and Wales, and prescribed the biomedical subjects and practical skills in which students needed to gain proficiency and so be granted registered nurse status by the GNC. Textbooks over the period of these syllabuses were tools used by training schools to impart the curriculum to student nurses for reaching the standard necessary for nurse registration. The system is explored in depth elsewhere (Bradshaw, in press).

This system of the nurse apprentice commanded nursing and nurse training totally for over a century. It may be the case that it still controls the image of the nurse in the public mind. A brief survey of its nature and ethos is essential to an understanding of what displaced it in 1979.

The national nursing syllabus for England and Wales 1923–1977

Developments 1919–1923

From the date of the Nurses' Registration Act in 1919, and the foundation of the General Nursing Council, it became a legal requirement that nurse training be standardized and systematized in England and Wales. This was achieved by the introduction of a national training syllabus and examination. Training for competence specified standards that were explicit, defined, achievable and measurable.

The draft for the first syllabus of subjects for examination was drawn up by the Education and Examination Committee of the GNC and built on the system of training nurses at St Thomas's Hospital since 1860, seeking to extend it widely as a national system. The recommendations from the committee, which were formally adopted, were as follows.

First, that a Schedule signed by the chairman and matron of the hospital or, in the case of poor law infirmaries signed by the medical superintendent and matron, was required from every nurse applying to enter the State Examination certifying that the applicant had passed through the educational curriculum prescribed by the Council and was of good character.

Second, that the subjects for examination should include anatomy, physiology, elementary science (including hygiene, bacteriology, sanitation), first aid, gynaecology, materia medica, dietetics, surgical nursing and medical nursing. Candidates were required to pass an examination on all these subjects included in the syllabus issued by the Council. The State Examination was concerned with written papers, a *viva voce* examination and an examination on practical nursing (*British Journal of Nursing*, 1921: 187–89).

The first *Syllabus of Lectures and Demonstrations for Education and Training in General Nursing* (GNC, 1923a) was issued by the GNC in 1923 although unlike the first *Syllabus of Subjects for Examination for the Certificate of General Nursing* (1923b) it would never become mandatory. This first syllabus of training, as it was called, began with an introduction which stated that the 1919 Nurses' Registration Act had vested authority in the Council to make rules requiring candidates for admission to the Register to have undergone prescribed training and possess a prescribed experience in the nursing of the sick.

The Council realized the value of lectures and demonstrations by medical practitioners and other experts on their special subjects, but attached great importance to lectures and teaching being given by fully trained nurses: matrons, sister tutors, ward sisters and so on. For it was they who would bring the 'true nursing outlook' gained by personal knowledge and practical experience (GNC, 1923a: 2). Also necessary were revision classes, correction of note books and personal supervision at all stages of training.

The examination was divided into two parts. The Preliminary Examination was to be taken by all probationers, at any time after the first year of training, whether training for the general nursing or the supplementary part of the Register (fever nursing, mental nursing, mental defective nursing, sick children's nurses). Anatomy and physiology, hygiene and the first part of the theory and practice of nursing were covered. The Final Examination for general nurses contained the remainder of the syllabus (first aid, gynaecology, materia medica, dietetics, surgical nursing and medical nursing), and the subjects mentioned in the Nurses' Chart.

The Nurse's Chart was to be retained by the nurse but marked by the teaching sister and deposited in the matron's office by the nurse at the conclusion of her work in each ward. It was a sheet of paper appended to the syllabus and marked into columns. The type of each ward (surgical, medical, children and gynaecology) was entered along the top. Downwards were detailed the various procedures in which the nurse was expected to become proficient. Examples of this were: domestic ward management, bedmaking and bedbathing, artificial feeding, enemas, injections, infusions, drug administration, dressings, and so on. The chart stated that it was drawn up as a suggestion by training schools. As the sister taught the nursing points she was requested to mark in the column descriptive of her ward (that is, whether it was medical, surgical, children's or midwifery or gynaecology). One stroke – / – was to signify that the nurse had been shown but was not proficient in the detail; two strokes crossed – × – indicated that the nurse had been taught and was proficient. The X was accompanied by the sister's initial.

Subsequent developments in the syllabus 1952–1977

Student nurses were prepared for practical and personal bedside hospital care. Although the syllabus changed in later decades to incorporate psychosocial knowledge and skill, and in relation to health promotion, specializing in district nursing or health visiting would occur only after initial state registration was achieved. Over the next decades the apprenticeship method of training, with its balance of biomedical knowledge, practical skill, and emphasis on personal character, was perpetuated in successive syllabuses. As it was updated it was gradually reformed. In 1952 the new syllabus separated the practical ward chart from the syllabus of subjects, and it became a more detailed stiff-covered book instead of a sheet folded at the back of the syllabus (GNC, 1952, GNC, undated). But there were no major changes, except for the introduction into the syllabus of two new subjects, human behaviour in illness and social aspects of disease. The syllabus was again revised in 1962. It had three main sections: the principles and practice of nursing including first aid; the study of the human individual; and concepts of the nature and cause of disease and principles of prevention and treatment. The record of practical instruction was altered to allow for more individual entries.

In 1969 the syllabus was again revised, and the record of practical instruction was now included in the syllabus (GNC, 1969). Subjects such as care of the paralyzed and dying were added, and the classroom-based practical examination, assessed by GNC examiners, was replaced by four ward-based practical assessments, assessed internally by the training school. The last syllabus published by the GNC in 1977 allowed for more individual interpretation, and removed the record of practical instruction and the need for external assessment by GNC examiners (GNC, 1977a,b,c,d).

The content of training: nursing textbooks informing the syllabus

For over a century, from the 1870s until the 1970s, four principles formed the foundation for the development of the good nurse. To this end, writers of nursing textbooks sought, first, to develop the moral character of the nurse. Second, they intended to equip nurses with the requisite knowledge and skill needed for their purpose of personal patient care. Third, they emphasized the method of learning as primarily by example of the ward sister. Fourth, they focused on relationships, both with colleagues and patients. These four categories will be used as a framework for the following analysis.

Developing the moral character of the nurse

The first principle of the traditional nursing system rested in the moral character of the nurse. One of the earliest nursing textbooks, included in the reading list for probationer nurses at St Thomas's Hospital, was by Florence Lees (1874), a superintendent who oversaw the care of the wounded in the Franco-Prussian War. Her experience in France and Germany was influenced by the religious nursing work of Roman Catholic sisters and Protestant deaconesses, and she saw the care of the sick in civilian life as occurring within this ethos. Lees's book was intended for nursing leaders, those in authority over nurses in training, especially the ward sisters. It described the practical knowledge that the nurse required, including bandaging, enemata, and prevention of bedsores.

In her introduction, Lees expanded on the purpose of nursing as the paramount duty of civilization concerning issues of life and death, and in which nurses were privileged to be involved. She listed the qualities nurses should learn in training school: cleanliness, neatness, obedience, sobriety, truthfulness, honesty, punctuality, trustworthiness, quickness and orderliness. The nurse was also to be patient, cheerful and kindly.

This introduction is typical. *Hints for Hospital Nurses*, published in 1877, was written jointly by two Nightingale nurses, Rachel Williams, of St Mary's Hospital, London and previously of Edinburgh Royal Infirmary, and Alice Fisher, of the Fever Hospital, Newcastle-upon-Tyne. Their textbook begins by entreating women not to enter nursing for love of notoriety, false sentiment, or even as just a means of earning a living. Nursing had to be an 'inborn love' of the work which was sadly given to only a few (Williams and Fisher, 1877: 1).

The Lady Superintendent of the Hospital for Sick Children, Great Ormond Street, Catherine Wood (c.1887) held to a similar position in *A Handbook of Nursing for the Home and the Hospital*. The nurse was not born but made, and required six qualities of character: presence of mind, gentleness of heart and thereby of touch, accuracy, memory, observation and forethought.

That care relied on a moral ethic was constantly repeated. Eva Lückes (1892, 1898), Matron of the London Hospital, asserted that the indispensable qualities of the vocation to nurse were self-discipline, personal responsibility for learning, truthfulness, obedience, punctuality, loyalty and the kindliness of genuine compassion. Any complaints against nurses were rarely about failures in practical duties: 'It is noteworthy that the grievance is almost always due to the lack of those personal qualities which are absolutely indispensable to real nursing' (Lückes, 1898: ix).

Such approaches to cultivating moral character predominated in textbooks written during the twentieth century. Esther Fisher, Matron of New End Hospital, Hampstead and author of *The Nurse's Textbook* (1937: 1), introduced her book by describing nursing as 'a sacred calling', its purpose being to alleviate the sufferings of humanity which should not therefore be taken up lightly. For this reason the qualities of the nurse were very important. A similar view was taken by Evelyn Pearce, a former Senior Nursing Tutor at the Middlesex Hospital, a Member of the GNC, and an Examiner in Nursing, Fever Nursing and Epidemiology for the Diploma in Nursing, London University. Her seminal nursing textbook, *A General Textbook of Nursing*, required reading for generations of student nurses, was published in 18 editions from 1937 to 1971. Pearce consciously saw nursing as evolving while maintaining the same ethos. By kindness and thoughtful sympathy, Pearce taught, fears could be dispelled. Patience, gentleness, tact, confidence and cheerfulness were displayed in the smallest acts of care.

Teaching technical knowledge and practical skill

The second principle of the tradition was the importance attached to biomedical knowledge and practical skill. Textbooks were designed to be practical. Their main focus was practical skill and theoretical knowledge of patients' conditions. Teaching of diseases and conditions was carried out by doctors, and many textbooks were written by them for nurses. The Nightingale School syllabus from its earliest days, for example, recorded Mr Croft's textbook (1873), as well as a manual by a surgeon at the Royal Devon and Exeter Hospital, Edward Domville (1885). Medical and surgical lectures given to nurses in training at Addenbrooke's by Laurence Humphry were published in 1889. The content included anatomy and physiology, diseases and their nursing, baths, enemata, poultices, bandaging and dietetics. The author acknowledged Sir Dyce Bryceworth's notes of lectures to probationers at St Thomas's Hospital, and Mr Croft's hints on nursing surgical cases. Wilfred Hadley, physician and pathologist at the London Hospital, lectured to nurses there, and wrote textbooks from these lectures (1902). Percy Lewis (1890), Honorary Medical Officer to the Victoria Hospital, Folkestone, wrote a textbook which embodied the course of instruction he gave in a series of lectures at the Salop and Southampton Infirmaries. In the twentieth century textbooks for nurses continued to be written and regularly updated by physicians and surgeons (for example, Toohey, 1953; Moroney, 1950; Sears, 1953). Nursing treatments reflected the contemporary scientific context (Voysey, 1905; Stewart and Cuff, 1899-1913; Ashdown, 1917–1943).

Training was to strengthen the qualities of the nurse, but not produce them: 'Examinations, at the best, can only demonstrate that the candidate has learnt enough to enable her adequately to exercise her profession; they can never prove that this or that woman is a good nurse.' (Stewart and Cuff, 1899:7; 1903:7; 1904:7; 1910:7; 1913:6). The essence of nursing was the patient, who must always be the nurse's first care. The nurse should be ever alert to anticipate his wants and needs. She could not go wrong if she 'always remembers the humanity of her patients, and makes their comfort and wellbeing her first thought . . . Her manner towards her patients should be characterized by dignity and gentleness' (Stewart and Cuff, 1899:8; 1903:8; 1904:8; 1910:8: 1913:6).

This textbook is particularly interesting for the insight it gives into the condition of patients at the turn of the century. In the chapter entitled 'Personal care of the sick', in all editions of the book, Stewart and Cuff describe how the nurse should wash the patient. The authors tell the nurse to change the washing water several times, implying that the patient might be very dirty. The face was washed first, the body being taken in small sections afterwards, each being carefully dried and covered with blankets. Hairwashing needed to take into account the likelihood that the patient's hair might be extremely dirty and infested. Responsibility for such care fell to nurses, from whatever rank or background.

According to Alice Dannatt, Lecturer on Domestic Hygiene and Honorary Superintendent of District Nursing and formerly Lady Superintendent of the Royal Infirmary, Manchester and Matron Superintendent of the Preston and County of Lancaster Royal Infirmary and Fever Hospital, the nurse needed to carry out the doctor's directions. She should learn to notice, 'without seeming to notice, the flush of feverishness, the beads of weakness, the expression on the face of pain, the shiver, that danger-signal that must at once be mentioned to Nurse or Sister'. She needed skill to manage the helpless patient; skill for minor surgical dressings; and much more besides. Training brought knowledge and, with it, confidence (Dannatt, 1893: 19–20).

This system was perpetuated in twentieth-century textbooks written by ward sisters, sister tutors and hospital matrons throughout the British Isles (for example, Oxford, 1900–1923; Riddell, 1914–1939; Vivian, 1920; Smith, 1929; Cochrane, 1930; Gration, 1944, 1946; Gration and Holland, 1950–1959). Over the decades, patterns changed but virtues did not.

A cogent example of this system is to be found in the writings of Evelyn Pearce. Bathing a patient meant that nurses could observe the patient and his condition, and record accurately what they could *see, hear, feel* and *smell*. Nursing observation was crucial from the point of admission until discharge. The keenness and interest of the student should never lapse into routine. Attention to detail, scrupulous care, thoughtfulness, structure and supervision were ever vital for good nursing. The methodical attention given to each limb during the bedbath, the carefully organized procedures of the hairwash and mouth care were to be rigorously observed. Each task followed an ordered procedure, maintaining the dignity of the patient throughout (Pearce, 1967: 28–37).

Pearce's prescription for the procedure of mouth care offers a vivid illustration. The reason and procedure for mouth care was detailed: why this was done, including conditions that affected the mouth. The patient was to be prepared and informed. Equipment was described and pictured laid up on a small tray. The bed should be protected, the mouth inspected 'and the treatment begun in some definite order'. Dentures were to be removed and brushed clean. The mouth was to be rinsed before being gently swabbed. The insides of the cheeks and the tongue needed special attention. All sordes and crusts should be gently removed. Each swab should be used once only (Pearce, 1967: 57–8).

The nurse's learning was graduated. She started in the classroom and ward with elementary knowledge of subjects such as hygiene and anatomy and physiology. She learned the more basic tasks of bedbathing, mouth care and bedmaking first. Her experience over the three years was gradually built up, the intention being to relate what she learned theoretically in the classroom to her practical experience on the wards. As she progressed she also advanced. She learned more complex diseases and their treatments and the nursing care procedures associated with them. As she was inducted into a tradition of practical care she learned to approach the human body with respect and sensitivity. The student nurse was expected to discuss and find reasons for what she was taught to do.

The role of the ward sister in the apprenticeship system of nurse training

The third principle of the traditional nursing system was the pivotal role of the ward sister. She was fundamental to passing on the moral tradition and spirit of nursing to student nurses personally. She inducted nurses into the tradition and ethos of care of which she was both guardian and custodian. The sister as the trainer, therefore, must not only exhibit moral qualities in her own person, but (which was much harder) must try to cultivate them in those placed under her, according to Lees in 1874.

In the nineteenth century it was recognized that good care signified good administration. The ward sister was responsible for the standard of nursing care on her ward. She was expected to have a detailed oversight of the ward, the needs and conditions of patients, and to manage the ward, including nurses, orderlies and domestic assistants. The hospital day was ordered with specified procedures and overseen by the ward sister. After breakfast patients were washed. 'Occasionally Sister has to remind her nurses of Miss Fisher's good advice: "Wash a patient as you would wish to be washed yourself." Whilst the washing progresses, Sister visits all her patients, observes their condition, and has a cheery good morning for each' (Dannatt, 1893: 23). Sister was expected to supervise all nursing practice, even in what might seem to be the minutest detail and ensure, for example, that beds were made without wrinkles because this might lead to bedsores. Prevention of these was crucial, noted Dannatt, because, as all ward sisters knew, once they arose they were very difficult to cure.

In the twentieth century, the central role of the ward sister in teaching and supervising nurses was still fundamental. Margaret Scales, former Ward Sister, Tutor and Night Sister at Guy's Hospital, and Tutor, Administrative Sister and Night Superintendent at Birmingham General Hospital and the Whittington Hospital explained the role in her *Handbook for Ward Sisters* (1952, 1958). The ward sister was the pivotal person on the ward. She was responsible for ensuring the friendly welcome to patients, and thoughtful attentions such as providing a newspaper, so that the patient would feel comfortable and secure. The ward sister should be sympathetic, genial, confident with a good memory, quick powers of observation, a lively imagination and attention to detail. She needed to know and understand each individual nurse; she should teach and maintain a careful supervision of all that happened on the ward. She needed to be a diplomat, an administrator and a decision-maker. She was also responsible for maintaining the community of the ward, and relationships with all those who visited the ward, including doctors, the almoner, the chaplain and so on.

According to Scales, a balanced mix of staff would ensure nursing and training standards could be maintained and so preserve a sense of law and order. Standard methods should be taught to avoid confusion. Routine procedures liberated the nurse from having to think about standard tasks, knowing that they were automatically taken care of, leaving the nurse free to attend sensitively to individual personal needs of the patient. Procedures and routines also ensured that a certain standard of care would be given to all patients by all nurses, as a basic safety net. If the nurse followed the particular procedure as a routine, then she could develop her own creative thinking, knowing the basics were fulfilled. The ward sister was responsible for supervising the practice of procedures. She was also responsible for teaching the nurse the principles underlying the procedures, and ensuring the nurse understood the reasons. As Scales argued, the Ward Sister wisely encouraged her nurses to put into practice the principles they learned during training. Questions should be encouraged and answered intelligently. Careless or slipshod work should not be treated leniently although understanding and help should be given.

Most importantly, the Ward Sister must know *how* to nurse and do so whenever the occasion arose. She was expected to be a practical person, rather than a deskbound theoretician. Vigilance should never be relaxed or purpose clouded, 'nor must "learning by experience" be the excuse for indifferent treatment by inexperienced nurses' (Scales, 1952: 23; 1958: 25). The hospital existed for the patient. The ward sister's role was to implement this in reality and bear the responsibility for so doing.

Professional etiquette: right relationships in the community of care

The authority of right relationships was the fourth principle advocated by the tradition. According to E. Margaret Fox (1912, 1914, 1924, 1930), Matron of The Prince of Wales's Hospital, Tottenham, hospital etiquette – courtesy in relationships between medical staff, patients, matron and ward sisters – enabled people of all classes to work together for the patient's well-being. This important assumption was born out by parliamentary evidence, which shows the extent to which this occurred in the everyday reality of hospital life at the end of the nineteenth century (House of Lords, 1890, 1891). All classes worked together. Williams and Fisher (1877), for example, were dismissive of suggestions of 'social embarrassment' made by those unfamiliar with hospital life.

Loyalty was the faithful allegiance to those in charge for the sake of the patient: 'Many important things are left to the judgement and faithfulness of the nurse to carry out unseen, unknown to any except her own conscience' (Fox, 1912: 475). Instructions should be carried out not only in spirit but by letter in order to gain the confidence of both doctors and patients. Even though doctors were human and liable to err, to be loyal to them did not imply servility. Fox expanded this approach in her textbook, *First Lines in Nursing* (1914), and further editions retitled *First Steps in*

Nursing (1924, 1930). It was reiterated through the decades (Houghton, 1938–1965, Clarke, 1971).

According to Evelyn Pearce, the personality of a hospital was largely dependent on the human contacts made through the goodwill and keen interest of the doctors and nurses who were 'the living spirit of the hospital' (Pearce, 1953: 90; 1963b: 91; 1969: 79). Far from advocating blind obedience, Pearce wrote: 'It is essential that the nurse–doctor relationship should enable the nurse to discuss her patients in this way, and a thoughtful medical officer will appreciate it' (Pearce, 1953: 95; 1963b: 96–97; 1969: 83–84). Each person was important as part of a team rather than as isolated and competing individuals. 'Each one accepts their responsibility in a common purpose – the welfare of mankind. The nurse acts as a sort of moral "prop", quick to notice any pull away from and direct it back again to the centre, the Patient' (Pearce, 1953: 94; 1963b: 95; 1969: 83).

This moral tradition was often termed 'etiquette', a concept used to convey right manner and behaviour. Dorothy Emmet, at one time Professor of Philosophy at the University of Manchester, identified 'professional etiquette' as a borderline away from 'professional ethics'. Drawing on the work of the sociologist Talcott Parsons, she argued that etiquette is necessary to maintain 'affective neutrality', the emotional detachment needed to safeguard the professional relationship from being affected by personal preferences which may cloud judgements (Emmet, 1986: 504). This notion of professional relationships meant that leaders with power were not expected to use their power to dominate others into submissiveness, but rather should seek to be aedificatory: to use their power to build up subordinates (Emmet, 1958: 284). The conception of 'professional etiquette' within nursing tradition precisely embodied Emmet's understanding.

The principles underlying the traditional nursing system: both profession and vocation

As nursing developed through the nineteenth and twentieth centuries it was conceived of as both a vocation and a profession. This conception was rooted in the origin of the word 'profess' in the sense of an outward demonstration of an inward conviction. As Nightingale had written:

> I must have moral influence over my Patients. And I can only have this by being what I appear – especially now that everybody is educated so that Patients become my keen critics and judges. My Patients are watching me. They know what my profession, my calling is: to devote myself to the good of the sick. They are asking themselves: Does that Nurse act up to her

profession? This is no supposition. It is a fact. It is a call to us, to each individual Nurse, to act up to her profession.

(Nightingale, 1888)

Therefore, nurse training under this system was not merely seen as the mechanistic passing of examinations, as important as this was, but it involved a strong personal and relational component. Ward reports and records of practical experience were tools by which the nurse was individually known to ward sisters and charge nurses, and also matrons. Personal interviews at regular intervals with ward sisters or charge nurses and notably matrons meant that the work, skills, knowledge and attitudes of the student nurse were closely and intimately monitored. Her report and record of instruction and practical experience were written and recorded by the ward sister and charge nurse in the nurse's presence and presented to the matron by the student personally.

Because training was to fit the nurse for a clearly defined purpose – the production of the bedside nurse, whose primary function was to care for the sick person – the knowledge and skill required of the nurse was carefully prescribed. The nurse learned her behaviour by example, particularly from the ward sister, as Lelean affirmed in her study of ward communications as late as 1975. The ward sister was the custodian and guardian of a tradition in which order, procedure, structure, self-discipline and supervision were key features. In this tradition competence was related to the nature of the nurse's role as a practical bedside nurse, generally in hospital, although community work was not thereby precluded. The moral character of the nurse, and the moral authority of right relationships underpinned this purpose.

Breaking away from vocation

Criticisms of the traditional nursing system of training

The British nursing profession was generally united in its core vocational values and practices until the 1960s. It was understood to be a body of people holding together a complex of formal knowledge and skills for the sake of service to the community. At its heart was an ethical covenant approach to work rooted in vocation (Bradshaw, 1994). Perhaps the most enduring symbol of this tradition was the bedpan, the receptacle for the patient's excrement, which nurses were taught to carry with pride as an emblem of service (*Nursing Times*, 1963: 281). It exemplified the vocational role of the nurse, on which all her complex training was built.

This ethical approach corresponded to definitions of 'professionhood' formulated by academic sociologists during the 1940s and 1950s

(Freidson, 1986). By the 1960s, however, the idea of a profession was viewed less positively by academics. It began to be seen as expertise sanctioning power for an élite which used the ethical orientation as an ideology to gain or preserve status and privilege (Freidson, 1986: 29). The social scientist Brian Abel-Smith appeared to take this viewpoint in his history of nursing published in 1960. He held that arguments over professional status were the expression of domination by the élite. The vocational attitude resting in a moral imperative of self-abnegation prevented the emancipation of the profession:

> Although the hours, the pay, and the attitude of management were out of line with the standards set by the world outside, nurses were deterred from vehement protest. They were restrained by the discipline which matrons had imposed on them, by their loyalty to their group and to their hospital, and by the spirit of uncomplaining service which was taken to be the heritage of their profession. Underfed, overworked, and underpaid, they struggled on rather than break a "professional" code of honour. Activism was unprofessional, worse still it would have undermined the cherished spirit of vocation: it smelt of hard bargaining and the pursuit of selfish material interests. It was also unfeminine.
>
> (Abel-Smith, 1960: 245).

Arguably Abel-Smith's analysis was supported by the work of the psychologist, Isabel Menzies (1960, 1961a, b, c, 1970). Menzies believed that the traditional system of nursing was a social defence system which represented the institutionalization of very primitive psychic defence mechanisms. A main characteristic of this system was that it facilitated the evasion of anxiety, and contributed little to its modification and reduction (Menzies, 1970: 38). The concept of nursing as a vocation of service was an idealization that repressed personal development. The nursing profession needed a new basis and a new status. This was in direct contrast to the view of the nursing examiner, teacher and author, Evelyn Pearce, one of the last representatives of the vocational tradition. In her revised book, *Nurse and Patient*, published at that time (Pearce, 1969: 72), Pearce argued that vocational service through work and not for self-interest alone is what gives it its value. Conditions and circumstances might change but nursing as nursing did not. It always demanded a certain degree of love, and essential sacrifice. It depended on unselfconsciousness (Pearce, 1969: 10). This was the very opposite to the position advanced by Menzies.

The profession itself became divided as secularism grew during that period. The Platt Report on nurse education, from the Royal College of Nursing (RCN, 1964), was criticized by the GNC (GNC, 1965). The vocational ethos of nursing was increasingly subject to question and criticism. Not all agreed that the valuable asset of vocation should be lost (Wyatt, 1978), but despite such cautions, by the 1970s the philosophical shift away from the vocational tradition was clearly discernible in the writings of two crucial nursing educationists. Barbara Fawkes, Chief Education Officer of the GNC (Fawkes, 1970, 1972) and Eve Bendall, from 1973, Registrar at the GNC (*Nursing Times*, 1972: 1403; Bendall, 1975, 1977) and in 1981 appointed Chief Executive Officer of the shadow English National Board for Nursing, Midwifery and Health Visiting (ENB, 1983), both advocated radical forms of change. Bendall's argument was that the nursing ideal did not correspond to reality.

The Briggs Report and a new professional status – education not training

In 1970 a review of nursing was set up by the government, under the chairmanship of the historian Asa (later Lord) Briggs. Changes in education were fundamental to the new professional status demanded of the nursing profession. The Briggs Report set out the case for a radical change in the system for preparing future nurses. The report recommended various organizational changes, as well as changes in education, and the setting up of Colleges of Health free to employ specialists who were not nurses (Report of the Committee on Nursing, 1972: 103–14, paras. 346–99). The report envisaged the building of links between nursing and administration and management on the one hand, and psychology, sociology and so on, on the other hand. It also recommended building links with professions allied to medicine, in particular, social services. Importantly, no explicit role for clinical doctors in nurse education was envisaged. Nurses would instead be taught by academic physiologists and biologists, who would probably not be clinical doctors.

The report proposed that the education of the nurse would no longer be standardized and universal. Service and education were to be very definitely separate. There were no longer assumed to be any inherited principles or tradition. This was the construction of a new kind of nurse. Nurse training in future should no longer be influenced by doctors. No longer instrumental in nurse training, the influence of doctors and their medical knowledge base would inevitably recede as a consequence. And, as he later said, Briggs (1979) was keen to bring into the nursing profession some of the ideas about methods of learning that were at work in the educational world as a whole.

Strangely, however, Briggs' main recommendations contradicted many nurses' opinions documented in the report. A majority of nurses and midwives who had recently trained rated both tutors' and doctors' teaching highly, and only a minority were unhappy with the quality of instruction on the wards from staff nurses and sisters (Report of the Committee on Nursing, 1972: 63–4, paras. 209–10). These opinions from grass-roots nurses were consistent with another study of student nurses in Oxford (MacGuire, 1966: 5d), which argued that a more academic nurse education would negatively affect nurse recruitment. Furthermore, abundant evidence from this period pointed to the fact that vocational values remained deeply held by many nurses and ward sisters, amongst whom there was a strong resistance to change (MacGuire, 1961; Marsh and Willcocks, 1965; Dutton, 1968; Singh, 1970, 1971a, b; Singh and MacGuire, 1971; Parry-Jones, 1971). Many ordinary nurses opposed any radical change. This evidence is examined elsewhere (Bradshaw, in press).

The 1979 Nurses, Midwives and Health Visitors Act: the final break with the apprenticeship tradition

Although it took seven years from the publication of the 1972 Briggs report to its implementation as the basis for the 1979 Nurses, Midwives and Health Visitors Act, these years consolidated the changing nursing ideology. According to Lord Briggs, speaking in 1983, the intervening years had seen profound changes. Some were economic, but some were within nursing itself, 'of trade unionism and attitudes which were not there in 1972' (Briggs, 1983: 8). The 1979 Act marked the decisive break with the apprenticeship tradition of nursing.

The Minister responsible for introducing the Bill to the House of Lords stated that the Bill was concerned with the reorganization of nursing bodies and a new unified structure which would look at training needs in the three professions (Wells-Pestell, in House of Lords, 19 February 1979b: 1643–52,). The Bill established a framework for formulating education and training of nurses for the future. It did not itself say what the future education and training should be, nor whether there should be any changes from what presently existed. It was limited to the creation of a framework within which these decisions could be made, and was there-fore about organizational change rather than the content of training. The future of the nursing profession was entrusted to the profession's leaders.

The provisions of the Bill were derived from the Briggs Report, and the recommendations and context of the report were summarized in the intro-duction of the Bill. The Briggs Report's emphasis on the continuum of education and training and the concept of the integrated statutory frame-work which flowed logically from it, was affirmed, but it was stressed that the Bill did not tackle questions of detailed changes. The Bill itself did not mean there would be changes in training, or that patterns of training would change overnight. The purpose of the Bill was to establish the United Kingdom Central Council for Nursing, Midwifery and Health Visiting, which would be responsible for registering practitioners and enforcing standards of professional conduct through the disciplinary process.

The Minister noted that while the professions had a major say in governing their own affairs, and in setting standards of education and training, others had an important contribution to make. He cited as examples medicine, because of its acknowledged 'close relationship' with nursing, and also education: 'those skilled in the field of education have an important part to play in formulating the way in which the professions' kind and standard of training are determined'. There would therefore be members representing both fields on the council.

For the first time, in 1979, the nursing profession became responsible for its own self-regulation: the prime purpose of the new body. Members of Parliament, and the government generally, expressed faith and confidence in the leaders of the nursing profession, and trusted professional self-regulation, as the debates in Parliament over the period of the introduction of the Nurses, Midwives and Health Visitors Act 1979 show (House of Commons 1978a–d); House of Lords, 1979a–f. So, for example, the Secretary of State for Health, Kenneth Clarke recognized that the proper training of staff was vital, but believed he could trust this to the profession (Clarke, 1983: 54). As he wrote to the Chairman of the UKCC a decade later, it was for the profession to regulate itself (Clarke, 1989).

Professional self-regulation was to have a profound effect on the nature of the doctor–nurse relationship, as the parliamentary debates began to make obvious. One of the key facets of the apprenticeship tradition had been the relationship between nurses and doctors. This was both clinical and educational. Doctors had an important input into nurse training; and ward relationships were regarded as crucial to teamworking for the benefit of patients. There was mutual respect and clarity of roles. The 1979 Act called this relationship into question, for what appears to be the first time. Instead of interdependence, nurses were to be independent.

In the House of Lords an eminent medical man expressed his concerns. Lord Smith spoke on the interdependence of the nursing and medical professions (Smith in House of Lords, 13 March 1979c: 504–08). He thought it was impossible to contemplate the organization of the training of the nursing profession other than in the context of the total care of the sick. Nursing and medicine were so interdependent because they had a common objective, not degrees or diplomas, not the intellectual satisfaction of examinations, nor the advancement of science for its own sake, but the best interests of patients. Modern medicine was ineffective without good nursing as modern nursing would be irrelevant except against the background of enlightened medicine. Nursing and medicine were linked together as no two other professions were. To ignore this close and key relationship was a serious omission from the Bill.

Lord Smith was concerned that medical representation on the council would be undermined if education and medicine as well as other fields were lumped together. He noted the argument that doctors should not be given a special and different position. But, in his view, in relation to the nursing profession they already were and always had been. As for the question of whether they should be in a privileged position, only one group should be privileged: the patients. Lord Smith advocated representation of a small number of doctors on the nursing council that was to be formed, but the Bill itself made no recommendations on such details as the composition of the council. There was a very strong feeling that the traditional help and co-operation that the medical profession had given nursing, and still sought to give, was being marginalized (Smith, in House of Lords, 13 March 1979c: 513).

In response, Lord Briggs argued that he regarded the doctor–nurse relationship to be a key relationship that went beyond education to conditions of work. But he also believed that numbers should not be laid down. In Lord Briggs's view the future improvement of nursing rested specifically and uniquely in nurse teaching. The role of the nurse tutor needed to change in terms of changes in medicine and 'changes in the nature of the educational system and the way in which this approaches the learning process' (Briggs, in House of Lords, 13 March 1979c: 513–14). The foundations for the future development of the nursing profession were laid here in an entirely new model for nursing.

Conclusion

Vocational values underpinned the apprenticeship tradition of training nurses for over a century, from the 1860s to the end of the 1960s. Under this tradition, the purpose of nursing had been perceived clearly to be bedside care and service to the patient. The system of training nurses for this purpose involved four key principles: the development of moral character; the building up of technical knowledge, practical skill, routine and procedure; the authority, influence and supervision of the ward sister, and the induction into professional etiquette of right relationships. These principles and values came under profound criticism during the 1960s.

Changes recommended by the Briggs Report in 1972 decisively broke the tradition and set in motion a nursing profession which had a radically different value system. By the end of the 1970s, the traditional system was considered to be no longer acceptable by those who were to shape the future of the profession, despite the fact that many nurses were content with it. Politicians trusted the professionals to manage their own profession. The leaders of the nursing profession set nursing on an entirely new course freed from the constraints of governmental control, vocational values and medical relationships. The four principles of the tradition were to lose their significance, and eventually their meaning. The change was fundamentally negative, for the leaders of the profession did not at that stage have proposals for a replacement system. Chapter 2 will examine the consequences of this break, and the new professional values and new system of education that came to fill the vacuum.

CHAPTER TWO

The autonomous practitioner – statutory and educational changes 1981–1986

Introduction

Following the passage of the 1979 Nurses, Midwives and Health Visitors Act, the apprenticeship tradition was gradually dismantled. The first half of the 1980s was the period in which the leaders of the nursing profession sought to redefine the profession in the light of its own autonomy. This involved a separation from the past, a severing of links with medicine and the medical model, and the search for a new educational direction. This chapter examines the thinking behind nursing developments in this period, from the Royal College of Nursing (RCN), the United Kingdom Central Council for Nursing, Midwifery and Health Visiting (UKCC), and, for reasons of depth and systematic analysis, the English National Board for Nursing, Midwifery and Health Visiting (ENB). England, therefore, may be seen as a representative example for the way legislation was implemented in the whole of the UK.

New nursing thinking: redefining nursing

Standards and structures

In 1981 the RCN published two documents, *A Structure for Nursing* and *Towards Standards* (RCN, 1981 a,b). David Rye, Director of Professional Activities at the RCN, and Sue Pembrey, a leading nurse who had been a member of the Briggs Committee, spoke to the Central Committee for Hospital Medical Services (CCHMS), composed of consultant doctors, about their significance (*BMJ*, 1982: 1130–32).

Rye opened the discussion by outlining concerns since 1978. These concerns involved problems of resources, increasing deficiencies in trained available nursing manpower, and service demands. There was felt to be a need to define good nursing care and to find ways to measure it. The possibility of producing indicators and developing a framework for the measurement of good nursing care, Rye argued, was now recognized to be an illusion.

Pembrey supported Rye's analysis and gave personal examples. As a ward sister on a surgical ward she discovered that nurses did not know what patients were eating at meals, their bowel function after bowel surgery, and were not able to control patients' pain because of the strict routine of drug rounds.

The reasons for such poor practice were analysed and were assumed to result from the lack of the individual nurse's responsibility and account-ability for individual patients. A minimum standard should be set for responsibility and accountability of the clinical nurse towards her patient. The RCN thought it important to effect a switch from too much reliance on external routines and rituals to personal responsibility; individual clinical nurses should see themselves as setting professional standards.

A Structure for Nursing (RCN, 1981a) sought to implement a single career pattern for nurses instead of the two-tier structure of training that had developed. A flatter management structure was advocated along with an opportunity to give proper priority to the clinical roles of nurses at all levels. *Towards Standards* (RCN, 1981b) suggested a move away from quantitative data to a more qualitative analysis of the individual nurse practitioner in a particular context. Two major principles were estab-lished: first, the concept of individualized patient care, and the ability of the trained nurse to be able to interpret and to develop within that philos-ophy; and second, the notion of accountability in clinical practice.

Towards Standards identified three factors as prerequisites for this development: the philosophy of nursing, the relevant knowledge and skills, and the notion of accountability. Poor practice was related to an inadequate conception of what nursing was. Nurses should see the patient as a whole, help the physician carry out a therapeutic plan to improve health, help the patient recover from illness or support him in death. Competence underpinned accountability and responsibility, and continu-ing professional development – currently lacking for 75 per cent of ward sisters – was crucial in keeping relevant knowledge and skills up to date.

In considering the nurse's individual responsibility for good standards of practice, Pembrey argued that more work was needed to identify patients' nursing needs and solve patients' problems. The nursing process sought to do this in a systematic way. Standards were not the responsibility of the management or the regulatory council but of the individual nurse.

The doctors' response

The consultants were not convinced by this new nursing direction. R. Hopkins thought that most consultants would want to recognize the importance of the clinical nurse and see her salary commensurate with her experience and responsibility. But the concept of autonomy concerned him if it indicated nurses would initiate paramedical services and therapies. To decide autonomously without the control of the consultant would lead to conflict.

E. B. Lewis was saddened by the document, in which he saw a nursing inferiority complex allied with a wish to expand the role of the nurse for self-aggrandizement rather than for the advantage of the team. Patients came into hospital under the care of the GP or consultant and not under the care of the nurse. All concerned were looking for a rise in standards and much should come from the recruitment of better educated and more academic nurses. Auxiliaries should be better trained, and there should be more liaison in such discussions between consultants and nurses.

While supporting proper pay for nurses, L. P. Harvey warned against the 'takeover' by nurse 'doctors', and the trouble this would bring. He wished that the RCN had had 'the common decency' to talk to consultants before trying to 'threaten and blackmail' them. A. P. J. Ross wondered whether the clinical nurse would accept this transfer of authority, accountability and responsibility, and the legal responsibility this involved.

In reply, Rye denied that nurses wanted to take over doctors' roles, but nurses were increasingly expanding their role by being delegated doctors' tasks. The nurse's legal responsibility concerned her nursing role and the nursing care she gave. The consultants' response was 'unbelievable' to Rye. Pembrey echoed Rye's reaction. Nursing care was complex and patients were admitted not only under the care of the consultant, but for nursing care. Nurses did not want to take over doctors' work but increasingly they were having to give intravenous drugs, undertake parenteral feeding and so on. Housemen expected them to do this. A nurse was responsible and accountable for her actions as well as for the care and comfort she gave.

W. J. Appleyard feared that nurses without clinical expertise would make decisions instead of consultants, and F. W. Wright said that many nurses to whom he spoke did not know who the senior nurse was. R. K. Greenwood wanted more 'battle-axe matrons' in uniform; there were not enough State-registered nurses. J. M. Cundy thought nurses should elect their own managers. D. Kenward had found the nursing process useful in his hospital. G. Cohen, however, disagreed and shared no enthusiasm for it. In his experience it made no difference to the nurse–patient relationship. The nurse would still have her day off, and therefore be away from the patient. He reflected that another unsatisfactory development over the years had been the taking away of nurse training from ward sisters into training schools.

In his conclusion to the debate, Rye made two comments. First, he affirmed the clear position of the RCN against industrial action. His second comment related to nurse training. The suggestion that nurses in training should be taken out of the clinical setting and put into universities was *not* a concept being floated by the RCN, he argued. The RCN wanted only separate funding for nurse education, to have it taken out of competition with service resources and classified separately. Less than three years later, in April 1985, the RCN Commission on Nursing Education would advocate the removal of nurse training from the clinical setting into colleges.

The nursing process

Many doctors had strong reservations about the direction being taken by the nursing profession. Their main concern was that nurses were encroaching on doctors' legal and medical responsibilities. A major communication gap appeared to open between the two professions on where the nursing leadership was taking nursing.

In 1983 the *British Medical Journal* reported a heated debate held by the Joint Consultants Committee about the 'nursing process' approach to nursing (*BMJ*, 1983: 439). The nursing process was the new method of organizing nursing care, drawn from North America, which individualized patient care into a process of assessment, planning, implementation and evaluation, controlled by the nurse. The consultants were unhappy about the lack of discussion with the medical profession, the increase in nurses' paperwork, and a rather general unease that nurses were attempting to shift the clinical management of the patient away from the medical profession and on to themselves.

The following year, the *BMJ* published a debate on the nursing process between a doctor, Professor J. R. A. Mitchell, and a nurse, Ray Rowden, which was later also published in *Nursing Times* (Mitchell, 1984a, b; Rowden, 1984a, b). Drawing on a contemporary textbook on the nursing process (McFarlane and Castledine, 1982), Mitchell expressed his doubts about the practical details of the process, and the nature of knowledge required by nurses at different levels of experience. He was also worried about the motivation of advocates of the nursing process. He believed it formalized a bid for nursing independence and autonomy and a removal of medical constraints, a concern of many doctors. Nurses were setting themselves against doctors, whom they felt had for too long held them subservient. They wanted to redefine their role.

Although Mitchell found some aspects of the nursing process concept praiseworthy, particularly the stated patient-orientated objective, he hoped that an informed debate would pre-empt any wide-scale introduction: 'No introduction without discussion and evaluation' (Mitchell, 1984a: 219). He saw the nursing process as a thesis that needed to provoke an antithesis. He hoped that this would lead to an informed debate after which an acceptable synthesis could be reached. Both at the beginning and end of his article he referred to Nightingale's concept of nursing. He argued that the debate should focus on the two key questions that Nightingale had identified: 'What is a nurse?' and 'How should nurses and doctors work together in the provision of patient care?' (Mitchell, 1984a: 219).

Rowden responded that the traditional image of nursing, presupposed by Mitchell, was now being challenged: 'The popular image of nurses as compliant and devoted flows from the misconceptions held about the history of the profession' (Rowden, 1984a: 219). Dismissing Nightingale, Rowden argued that Ethel Bedford Fenwick was the real influence on the shape of academic, modern nursing, which he defended (Rowden, 1984a: 220). Rowden was confident in the revolutionary nature of change.

The new way of thinking about nursing education was articulated by Baroness McFarlane, at the time Professor and Head of Department at the University of Manchester, Chairman of the shadow ENB (ENB, 1983), and a key proponent of the nursing process. She argued that previous nursing syllabuses had been a pale reflection of the medical curriculum; they dealt with body systems and diseases. Much of this was redundant knowledge because it was irrelevant and neglected the emerging body of nursing knowledge. However, what followed in the nursing curriculum were curriculum fashions: the use of dialectical themes such as human development or 'total patient care', and more recently, a problem-solving approach, were phases that were passed through. In McFarlane's department the focus was patient problems: 'As yet I see no sign of a coherent organizing framework in the statutory syllabus' (McFarlane, 1985: 269).

McFarlane referred to the doctoral and masters' studies by nurses in her department as providing the evidence for contemporary weaknesses in nursing. Progress in areas such as teaching communication and interpersonal relationship skills, according to McFarlane, was limited by hours available and teacher adequacy. Time for consolidation of practice in acute and general settings was sacrificed for breadth and variety. There was no structure for post-registration training and advanced clinical roles: 'There are no doubt advances, but how far have we progressed in the adequate preparation of nurses, even at basic level, for patient care?' McFarlane was calling for a multi-disciplinary college-based education for nursing. But she had clear intentions towards the limits:

What I am not advocating in the first instance is a move to higher education for the purpose of becoming a totally graduate profession. I am advocating a different kind of learning community with a multi-disciplinary faculty and strong research base and the ability to move between diploma and degree level work.

(McFarlane, 1985: 270)

She was keen to develop for nursing 'a learning community' that fostered 'self-actualization and flexible and creative behaviours'. This, according to McFarlane, would not occur in teacher-centred and didactic environments.

The changed syllabus for nurse education: legislation, regulation and competencies

Problems with nursing education were now surfacing arguably as a consequence of the less structured approach to nurse training introduced by the GNC in the 1970s. Cox, Lewin, Hewins and Bowman (1983) conducted a study on clinical learning in the early 1980s. As part of this study students' nursing skills, in the giving of a bedbath and the performance of aseptic technique, were observed and found wanting. In some cases the situation was positively dangerous. The problem was the lack of supervision that could correct students' mistakes. There was virtually no formal ward teaching, and teaching while doing was sporadic. Trained staff often missed opportunities to teach by working together, or by not initiating teaching when the ward was quiet. The principle of apprenticeship was violated because supervision, when it occurred, tended to be from other trainees rather than trained nurses.

The authors recommended a core clinical skills curriculum which would require all students to demonstrate competence in a specified range of nursing skills and responsibilities. While this might be thought to be turning the clock back to the previous system of ward-based assessments, the authors thought that a compromise could be reached with modern educational methods. A core clinical curriculum would be compatible with current nursing theory. The vital aspect of technical competence would then be integrated with the interpersonal aspects of nursing care.

For Marjorie Gott (1984), however, nursing practice in the wards was different to nursing practice as taught in school. The school emphasized the 'right' idealized way but rarely instructed or showed nurses how alternative practices could be performed in working reality, or warned nurses of the gap that would face them between the ideal and the real. There were tensions between bureaucratic behaviour, expected on the wards, and professional behaviour, expected in the school (even from bureau-cratically-minded teachers). Task allocation was considered to produce fragmented care and to be associated with bureaucratic behaviour. Patient allocation, which Gott recommended, was considered to be associated with professional behaviour. Teaching methods were traditional, mainly by lecture, and, in Gott's view, were ineffective in teaching skills, either practical nursing or social skills. Indeed, social skills, which were not a stated curricular goal, particularly needed improvement, she believed. Gott recommended progressive educational methods, which were student-centred rather than teacher-centred. She saw trained ward nurses and ward sisters as key learning resources, and recommended joint teaching/service appointments.

Many of these ideas, espoused by Gott, seem to have infused the new system of education. Statutory Rules brought in under the Nurses, Midwives and Health Visitors Act 1979 in 1983, introduced an entirely different approach to nurse training: regarded henceforward as 'educa-tion' rather than 'training'. This was built on the idea of 'competencies', but as will be seen, the interpretation of competence was rather different to that of Cox et al. (1983).

New legislation, 1983

The Statutory Instrument made under the 1979 Nurses, Midwives and Health Visitors Act, Nurses, Midwives and Health Visitors Rules Approval Order (1983) No 873, required courses leading to qualification for admis-sion to Parts 1, 3, 5, or 8 of the register:

> to provide opportunities to enable the student to accept responsibility for her professional development and to acquire the competencies required to:–
>
> (a) advise on the promotion of health and the prevention of illness;
> (b) recognise situations that may be detrimental to the health and well-being of the individual;
> (c) carry out those activities involved when conducting the comprehensive assessment of a person's nursing requirements;
> (d) recognise the significance of the observations made and use these to develop an initial nursing assessment;
> (e) devise a plan of nursing care based on the assessment with the co-operation of the patient to the extent that this is possible, taking into account the medical prescription;
> (f) implement the planned programme of nursing care and where appropriate teach and co-ordinate other members of the caring team who may be responsible for implementing specific aspects of the nursing care;

(g) review the effectiveness of the nursing care provided, and where
     appropriate, initiate any action that may be required;
(h) work in a team with other nurses, and with medical and para-medical
     staff and social workers;
(i) undertake the management of the care of a group of patients over a
     period of time and organize the appropriate support services;

related to the care of the particular type of patient with whom she is likely
to come in contact when registered in that Part of the register for which the
student intends to qualify.
> (Statutory Instruments 1983 No 873, The Nurses, Midwives and
> Health Visitors Rules Approval Order, Rule 18: 10)

As the rule continued, courses leading to a qualification for admission to
Part 2, 4, 6 or 7 of the register should be designed to prepare the student
to undertake nursing care under the direction of a person registered
under Part 1, 3, 5 or 8 of the register 'and provide opportunities for the
student to develop the competencies' required to assist in carrying out
comprehensive observation of the patient and help in assessing care
requirements; develop skills in assisting in the implementation of nursing
care; accept delegated nursing tasks; assist in reviewing the effectiveness
of nursing care; and work in a multi-disciplinary team.

To be registered under Parts 1–8 of the register, the student should:

(a) have her name on the index of students maintained by a Board; and
(b) have completed the relevant training required under rules 14 and 17
    of the rules; and
(c) have passed an examination, held or arranged by a Board in accord-
    ance with 6 (1) (c) of the Act:

which may be in parts, and which shall be designed so as to assess the
student's theoretical knowledge, practical skills and attitudes and demonstrate her ability to undertake the relevant competencies specified in rule
18 of these rules.
> (Statutory Instruments 1983 No 873, The Nurses, Midwives and
> Health Visitors Rules Approval Order, Rule 19 (1) (a) (b) (c): 11)

Cox et al. (1983) had wanted clearly specified core competencies. These
were not defined in the Act, except in the most general of terms, to allow for
a variety of interpretations. What had been so important for apprenticeship
training, – that is, a national syllabus which rigidly prescribed the content and
standard of scientific knowledge, technical skill and moral attitude, in terms
that were specific, explicit, and assessable – was entirely abandoned.

The Statutory Instrument became the basis for the *Syllabus and Examinations for Courses in General Nursing Leading to Registration in Part 1 of the Register* (ENB, 1985a). This was sent to chief nursing officers and directors of nurse education. In the accompanying letter the ENB described the syllabus as guidelines, developed for Schools of Nursing to assist translation from the existing syllabus to a curriculum. Since the syllabus was no longer printed in rules, the ENB stated, greater flexibility was possible. The Board had also considered many useful comments received on the devolution of the written examination and had made alterations in line with the comments.

Breaking up the common syllabus: flexible nursing education

In the introduction the ENB stated its original intention to revise the existing syllabus for courses leading to Part 1 of the professional register, but recognized that a major revision was inappropriate at that time. The guidelines were intended to assist individuals and groups wanting to translate the existing syllabus into a curriculum which, it was stated, would fulfil the needs of students and institutions within a varied and changing social and economic structure (ENB, 1985a).

This began, and indeed encouraged, the fragmentation of the common syllabus. The ENB believed that the 'agreed philosophy for nurse education within each individual institution will influence the development of the curriculum; it is therefore probable that there will be many interpretations'. Each curriculum planning team must agree the philosophy or statement of beliefs endorsed by the institution. From this the aims of the course would be developed.

While the ENB recommended freedom of interpretation in the curriculum there was less flexibility over teaching methods. In order to facilitate maximum learning it was appreciated that a wide variety of teaching methods must be employed. However, the ENB believed that students should be encouraged to adopt a self-directed approach to learning with opportunities to progress at their own pace to meet their own individual needs. In order to achieve this the ENB thought it helpful to consider methods of determining the student's level of knowledge and experience from which individualized programmes could be developed.

According to the ENB, there were many ways in which knowledge, skills and attitudes could be linked, dependent on local factors. The present syllabus identified certain essential nursing skills and procedures. The guidelines reflected a change in emphasis from task-orientation to patient-centred care and encompassed the competencies stated in the Nurses' Rules. The syllabus was comprised of three sections, A, B and C, which were not to be seen as separate entities 'but as threads which may be interwoven to create a complete curriculum' (ENB, 1985a: 1).

Each section was underpinned by the relevant clause from rule 18. Section A, 'Nursing Studies', was the theoretical foundation for nursing practice. This included concepts of health and theories and models in nursing. Behavioural sciences were detailed, and were to include psychology: the relevance and importance of psychology to general nurses in the maintenance of health, concepts of general psychology – cultural differences, communication and interpersonal skills, deprivation and loss, developmental psychology – human growth and development and sexuality, social psychology of the family, and sociology. (ENB, 1985a: 4).

Section B, 'Clinical Nursing Studies', was to include data collection, assessment, recording and disseminating information, planning, implementation and evaluation (ENB, 1985a: 7). Section C, 'Professional Studies', included social policies, organization and system supporting the development and practice of nursing. Under this section was the development of nursing, aspects of economics, health service studies, professionalization of nursing, research studies, teaching studies, management studies and legal and administrative studies, (ENB, 1985a: 9). This syllabus, intended as a guideline, and without mention of any practical clinical nursing skills, appears to have been very provisional because the following month the ENB produced a discussion paper of new proposals.

The supernumerary nurse: no longer marching 'to the drumbeat of service'

The mid-1980s saw three highly influential reports, the RCN Commission on Nursing Education (RCN, 1985a), the English National Board Proposals (ENB, 1985b) and the UKCC Project 2000 (UKCC, 1986a), which would have the revolutionary impact on nurse preparation that the English National Board had commended but not yet instigated. All three reports looked to place nurse education in higher education and recommended that the student nurse should have supernumerary and student status. No longer should she learn through apprenticeship. As the RCN report argued, students should no longer be overworked 'pairs of hands' whose own learning needs were secondary because they marched 'to the drumbeat of service' (RCN, 1985a: 8–9, para.1.6).

The RCN Commission proposals

The report published by the RCN Commission on Nursing Education in 1985 called for nursing education to be based in higher education. The nursing profession 'was, and is, gravely concerned about problems

inherent in the training and education of its members' (1985a: 7). While
admitting that the profession itself has been divided about the nature and
the cure of these problems, the report proposed radical reform.

The problems inherent in the training and education of nurses,
although not new, were now urgent. Previous solutions had been mere
palliatives, because hitherto 'nurses themselves have not agreed either
upon their nature or upon their cure'. Nothing less than fundamental
reform could now be effective. The changes that were proposed would
appear to many as 'dangerous and threatening, but should not (for that
reason alone) be rejected. Failure to undertake radical changes will, in any
case, be even more dangerous' (RCN, 1985a: 7, para. 1.1).

The Commission specified its reasoning. Large numbers of student
nurses posed problems of supervision for trained staff (RCN, 1985a: 8–9,
paras. 1.4–1.8). Nurses needed a broader curriculum and to learn
sociology and psychology (RCN, 1985a: 9–10, paras. 1.9–1.10). Teaching
was 'superficial and unconvincing' and the educational atmosphere was
'reminiscent of a 19th century teachers' training college rather than a
modern establishment of post-secondary education' (RCN, 1985a: 10,
para. 1.11). There was an 'often ill-articulated and ambiguous' demand for
'student status' which demonstrated an imprecise discontent (RCN,
1985a: 10–11, para. 1.12). But it also involved prediction and prophecy.
The standard of entry qualification for student nurses, which in 1983
involved 90 per cent of students on RGN courses having five or more O
Levels, would not continue, the report argued: 'Young people of this
quality will simply not continue to present themselves unless the present
institutional arrangements change' (RCN, 1985a: 11, para. 1.13). Student
nurses were bound to demand their rights for increased status (RCN,
1985a: 11–12, para. 1.14).

The final point was supported with evidence. It claimed that there was
a 15–20 per cent drop-out rate of the 24,477 students who entered
training, and a further 30 per cent would fail to meet qualification criteria
(RCN, 1985a: 12, para. 1.15). It was necessary to attract applicants into
nurse education who had adequate educational qualifications, as well as
personal attributes, and to hold them 'although not necessarily in their
present numbers' (RCN, 1985a: 12–13, para.1.16).

Yet statistics collected for the RCN Commission on recruitment and
wastage did not in themselves justify any radical changes in nursing education (Hutt, Connor and Hirsh, 1985; RCN, 1985b). What the Commission
wanted was a total change of ethos even though it knew well that its
proposals would meet hostile criticism: 'Even the most hostile critics of
change (and some of them will certainly make themselves audible in

public and private responses to this Report) will concede that patients are people . . .' (RCN, 1985a: 10, para.1.10).

The tone of the report was defensive. It advocated a change with which many, it knew, would disagree. The lay public did not believe there was anything wrong with nursing:

> One initial difficulty must be openly acknowledged. The layman will need to be convinced that anything very much is wrong. He is likely to believe that the nurse in our society may indeed be undervalued and underrewarded, but not that she is irresponsible or ill-prepared. His experience suggests that the public has confidence in the quality of practical nursing, and prompts the question "If the system of training is wrong, why are the products so good?" He will, moreover, be disposed, in a spirit of traditional Anglo-Saxon pragmatism, to favour a system which embeds training in practice and eschews fancy notions or theories of "Education". He will be sceptical of any attempts to move the training of nurses from its present base. He will, if pressed, want his bedside nurse to be trained and practical rather than educated and questioning. He will certainly not wish to be cared for after an operation by an amateur psychologist or (still worse) sociologist. Told that nurses learn their craft by being engaged from the beginning in the delivery of care, he will grunt his heartfelt approval.
>
> (RCN, 1985a: 7, para. 1.2)

Although the RCN Commission openly acknowledged that the layman would not want the change in the way nurses were educated, it asserted that most nurses and student nurses would welcome this change. But the report gave no evidence to substantiate this opinion.

Had ordinary nurses' attitudes changed so radically since the evidence produced by researchers such as MacGuire, Morton-Williams and Berthoud a decade earlier? This assertion was not only contradicted by the SCPR survey of nurses' opinions (Morton-Williams and Berthoud, 1971a, b), as well as the work of MacGuire (1961 and 1966) but also by evidence documented in the Briggs Report (Report of the Committee on Nursing, 1972) itself.

On the contrary, research studies (for example, MacGuire, 1961 and 1966) showed that nurses wanted a practical training at the bedside. If anything, as the SCPR study indicated (Morton-Williams and Berthoud, 1971a), nurses were most worried about weaknesses in the area of clinical teaching. While there was plenty of practice, there was a distinct lack of practical instruction. The same study demonstrated that nurses were very happy with the quality of their lectures, and the balance between theory and practice, although there were criticisms about timing that resulted from the 'block system': too much information compressed into too short a time. Although some tutors were subject to criticism, 'more often there was praise for tutors; they taught well, they answered questions carefully, and on the whole were excepted from the fairly harsh personal criticism often levelled at other senior nursing staff by students and pupils. In fact many students felt that they could approach their tutors if they had a particular grievance against a ward sister' (Morton-Williams and Berthoud, 1971a: 9).

The Commission chairman, Harry Judge, originally held the same view as the lay public. Responding to the criticism that he was biased – a higher educationalist wanting to move nursing into higher education – he admitted that before he began chairing the RCN Commission he himself believed that a move into higher education would be destructive for nursing. As he wrote in the *Nursing Times*:

> I have been told that somebody like me, working in a university, could have been expected to make a fuss about higher education. Nothing could be further from the truth. When I began to work with the commission, my prejudices all ran (*sic*) the opposite direction. I was the typical layman, convinced that higher education could only make a mess of something that was good in its own special way. Higher education has already had a lot of practice in doing that. But the evidence and the arguments convinced me that the other two major reforms – an improved course and supernumerary status – would not come about without the move into higher education.
>
> (Judge, 1986: 31–2)

Judge argued that evidence and argument changed his 'common sense' lay perception, yet he gives no references for either the evidence or argument that convinced him to change his mind. Indeed, the evidence ought to have reinforced his original opposition to changing nursing. Judge regretted the UKCC decision not to move nursing wholesale into higher education. He was not happy with nurses having merely a specialized 'advanced' nursing education. Rather he wanted nurses to have an all-round liberal education that would qualify them for jobs other than nursing.

English National Board proposals

In England, the ENB published its *Professional Education/Training Courses: Consultation paper* in May 1985, (ENB, 1985b) one month after the production of its new syllabus (ENB, 1985a). It seems that it wanted a more radical strategy than merely revising syllabuses. The letter from the Chairman, Audrey Emerton, that accompanied the document described the document as 'a strategy for change in the initial courses for nurses, midwives and health visitors'. Preliminary discussions had taken place with the Department of Health and Social Security and with the Department of Education and Science. These would need to be followed up. The recent publication of the RCN Commission on Nursing Education was seen as a welcome initiative. The ENB was hoping that its proposals would be seen as a 'more meaningful' preparation for nurses, midwives and health visitors, and would contribute to the work of Project 2000 by the UKCC.

The consultation paper was devised in the light of the 'crisis today' (ENB, 1985b: 4). Education was difficult because of the worker status of students, the throughput of patients in acute hospitals, conflict between European Community Directives and service needs, and the dilemma of a 'nursing model' curriculum in a medically structured environment. Added to this was a continuing fall in recruitment in mental nursing and mental handicap nursing, which themselves required more community nursing educational experience, and problems in shortcomings of paediatric nursing education, direct recruitment into midwifery, problems of recruitment in health visiting and the increasing recruitment of community nurses who were not district trained (ENB, 1985b: 4–5).

The ENB proposals presupposed a model of nursing that concentrated on health promotion and disease prevention: the nurse professional was expected to help and teach people to manage their own health effectively, with a particular focus on the community. The traditional concept of nursing as caring for the sick was more marginal. Nursing was envisaged as becoming a complex and sophisticated activity (ENB, 1985b: 9). The curriculum was designed to fit these presuppositions.

The Board's proposals were, broadly, for a common core initial training followed by qualification in specialisms, supernumerary status for students, collaborative links between health service institutions and higher or advanced further education institutions, preparation in both hospital and community for mental nursing, mental handicap nursing and paediatric nursing, programmes of post-initial education and a single category of nursing teacher.

As to course structure, it was proposed that the first year should be theory-centred, with student-centred learning and teacher-led practical placements. Subjects could include health promotion and maintenance, nursing theories and models, biological sciences, behavioural sciences, social policy and administration, epidemiology, information technology and liberal studies. The second year would be application-centred, notably, with supernumerary practice, and the third year, practice-centred and salaried.

The ENB consultation paper invited responses on a detailed question-naire included with the document. These were to be considered at the September meeting of the ENB and it does not appear they were published. In any event, the UKCC proposals appear to have overtaken the ENB.

The purpose of new nursing education

The clear assumption behind the change in nurse education was that nurses would benefit *qua* rounded and developed individuals rather than *qua* patient carers. In this sense then the focus was on nurses rather than nursing or patient care. The report *Implications for the Costs of Nurse Training in the U.K. of Changes in Learner Status* (Goodwin and Bosanquet, 1985), referred to in the annexe of research studies for the RCN Commission, reflected this paradox. The aim was to produce nurses who were more managerially capable – echoing the preoccupation of the earlier reports by Salmon (Ministry of Health Scottish Home and Health Department, 1966) and Briggs (Report of the Committee on Nursing, 1972):

> We do not assess the relative "quality" or "output" of RNs trained under the alternative systems [school of nursing, diploma and degree]. However, there seems to be consensus of opinion suggesting that the proposed system, by being geared to a greater extent towards the educational needs of the students and to a lesser extent towards the day-to-day manpower requirements of DHAs, would provide a "better" all round education and training in ward management (and nursing generally) than exists at present. The greater level of satisfaction student nurses would feel under the proposed system might lead to a reduction in the wastage rate during training (and so a reduction in the cost of training a RN).
>
> (Goodwin and Bosanquet, 1985: 208)

Whether patient care would be improved was a moot point, but the programme costs 'would have to be justified as an investment in an enhancement of nursing education and quality of care' (Goodwin and Bosanquet, 1985: 257).

In their recommendations to strengthen nurse education and separate it from practice, the ENB and RCN reports were similar. As Dingwall, Rafferty and Webster point out (1988: 223): 'Both tend to emphasize the benefits to nurses rather than discussing standards of care or patient welfare.' There was also a possible weakening of the professional control over the curriculum. Indeed in the ENB's proposals there was very little of specifically nursing content.

Also important was the motivation behind the reports. Dingwall et al. (1988) suggest that Harry Judge, Director of the Department of Educational Studies at Oxford, who chaired the RCN Commission, may have primarily been interested in providing students to fill higher education places. This point was also made by Jamie Fleming (1985: 54), in an interview with Judge. Fleming asked Judge whether the movement to higher education was 'a ploy to prevent colleges of higher education closing under the proposals of education secretary Keith Joseph?' Judge denied this, claiming he was concerned with strengthening the nurse's professional responsibility and competence through increased autonomy and accountability. In Judge's view all that was needed was for the government to transfer resources and then 'we'll discover first whether higher education wants nurses and, second, whether nurses want higher education' (Fleming, 1985: 54). But, as evidence to the UKCC shows, this second question – whether nurses wanted higher education – was dubious.

United Kingdom Central Council proposals

The UKCC Project Group, under a Project Officer, the sociologist Celia Davies, had published consultation papers in 1985 (UKCC, Project Papers 1–6,1985a, b, c, d, e, f), before publishing its report. These were published in *Senior Nurse* between November 1985 and January 1986, and in *Nursing Times* (UKCC, 1986a: 3). The report *Project 2000: A New Preparation for Practice* (UKCC, 1986a) was published in 1986. That same year, Project Paper 7 (UKCC, 1986b) entitled *Project 2000: The Project and the Professions: Results of the UKCC Consultation on Project 2000* described the 2,500 submissions mostly from the professional organizations as giving only qualified approval. Project Paper 8 (UKCC, 1987a), which considered costings, and Project Paper 9: Project 2000: The Final Proposals (UKCC, 1987b), were published the following year.

The UKCC Project Group reported in 1986 (UKCC, 1986a). Members of the group included nurse educationalists, directors of nursing as well as members outside nursing including three educationalists and an educational psychologist. As will be seen, there were criticisms that there were no practical clinical nurses on the committee, and no representatives from the medical profession. The report stated the case for change based on four main points. The current system was educationally deficient; it was disadvantageous for the service; it had led to recruitment problems; and it brought frustration within the profession.

In considering the first point, the report noted the volume of research literature which raised questions over existing educational techniques for teaching and learning and preparation for competence. These questions were themselves rooted in a particular philosophical stance that marked educational theory of that period, and which appears to have influenced the UKCC. Directly quoting the RCN Commission report quoted earlier, the UKCC criticized the poor conditions of service for teaching staff that 'conspire to generate an educational atmosphere reminiscent of a 19th century teachers' training college rather than a modern establishment of post secondary education' (UKCC, 1986a: 9–10, para. 1.12; RCN, 1985a: 10, para. 1.11).

Although there was wastage and dropout from courses, this should be viewed cautiously in any argument for change, the UKCC said. Best available recruitment and wastage figures provided by Hutt, Connor and Hirsh (1985) for the RCN Commission showed a lower dropout rate from courses than in the 1970s, and another recent study by Poulton (1985) showed an even smaller percentage of losses from training programmes in England and Wales. Moreover, there was further wastage from those who failed to pass examinations (UKCC, 1986a: 10, para. 1.13).

Nevertheless, like the RCN, the UKCC was concerned about educational quality and mode, the service/education compromise, and the current system that was so closely linked to service that it isolated the majority of students and staff from broader fields of education (UKCC, 1986a: 10, paras. 1.15–1.16).

The second point, disadvantages from the service standpoint, was similar to the RCN Commission criticism that the needs of the learner were subordinated to the needs of service. Students were being depended upon to provide the labour in a system of constant replacement for the wastage of trained staff. The present pattern was a 'collision course' because the needs of students clashed with service requirements (UKCC, 1986a: 11–12, paras. 1.18–1.23).

The third point concerned the problems of recruitment. This would seem to follow on from the previous point, the wastage of qualified nurses. But, in fact, the RCN study by Hutt et al. admitted that it was extremely difficult to record wastage rates of qualified nurses because there was no national source of data (Hutt et al., 1985: 137–138, para. 6.7). Nevertheless, it appears from manpower statistics, prepared by Brian Moores and given in the appendix of the UKCC report (UKCC, 1986a: 82, 87, fig. II.ii), that the percentage contribution of qualified staff increased in the previous decades, while from 1962 the number of students had declined. What concerned the UKCC in relation to recruitment was the 'demographic time bomb' and a declining pool of 18-year-olds (UKCC, 1986a: 12, para. 1.24). However, as the UKCC admitted, analysis of recruitment and wastage was complex and did not provide a cogent argument for change.

This leads to the final point, frustration within the profession. In the course of 40 meetings throughout the UK, the UKCC argued, there were criticisms of initial nurse preparation. These criticisms centred on the gap between theory and practice, fragmentation, divisions and overlap between different programmes and a lack of progression. Health visitors, district nurses and midwives criticized initial nurse preparation as 'rigid' and 'didactic'. According to the UKCC not all criticisms were from teachers but came from managers too. There was a 'threefold prescription for change'. The demand was for 'student status', a 'single grade of nurse' and, on occasions, 'a shift of all education into colleges of higher and further education'.

The report did not detail from whom these comments came, or how universal this demand was. Indeed, the Project Papers, which were expected to form the basis of this report, showed that many grass-roots nurses were not in support of change. There was not unqualified support for the UKCC proposals. At the end of Project Paper 7 consideration was given to the responses of 'today's students' (UKCC, 1986b: 24). Letters from Learner's Councils, from set representatives, from groups, usually of second and third year students, and from individuals were the most negative towards the new proposals. Their main worry concerned the level of practical experience that students would have once they became supernumerary. One student had asked, 'Why jettison the present system for an untried and unproved alternative?' Concerns were also expressed that inadequate funding might lead to a deterioration in standards of care. Costs and adequate staffing were also issues, as was 'the need for practical "hands-on" experience and fears that an "Americanized" and "academic nurse" could be the outcome of the proposals' (UKCC, 1986b: 26).

The writers of this Project Paper 7 (presumably under the Project Officer, Celia Davies) suggested that student responses contained misconceptions. They rejected as misconceptions statements from students that proposals would lead to a 'two year college programme' and involve 'two years of theory' and 'two years of health education'. They also disagreed with the rhetorical question of another student, who asked: 'Could we train a carpenter successfully if he never got to run his hands over a piece of wood for two years?' (1986b: 24). Such comments were considered by the authors of the Project Paper to be misguided, and were dismissed as not reflecting the theory and practice emphasis in the Report. Indeed, the authors of the Paper thought that they were the result of people reading only the summary. Yet, importantly, these comments did seem to reflect a more generalized grass-roots disagreement with Project 2000 proposals. An opinion poll for *Nursing Times* published in 1986 found that only 16 per cent of nurses interviewed thought the UKCC proposals were good or very good (Wilson-Barnett, 1986a; Kratz, 1986).

Nevertheless, the UKCC members were adamant about the need for radical change: 'It is clear, however, that things are felt to be wrong, and lowered morale and fears about standards are themselves further arguments in the case for change' (UKCC, 1986a: 12–13, paras. 1.27–1.29).

Against the background of a changing world the UKCC recommended that there should be a new registered practitioner competent to assess the need for care, provide care, and monitor and evaluate care, in institutional and non-institutional settings. A common foundation programme should underpin branch programmes for the various specialities. There should be a new, single list of competencies applicable to all registered practitioners at the level of registration and set out in the Training Rules. Students should be supernumerary to NHS staffing establishments throughout the period of training. A new helper grade would be monitored by the registered practitioner. Teachers should have opportunities for further training and full participation in wider educational activities. The practitioner of the future should be a 'knowledgeable doer' and a 'networker'(UKCC, 1986a: 40–41, paras. 5.18–5.24).

The competent nurse would be able to identify factors which affect physical, mental and social well-being; identify social and health implications of physical and mental handicap, pregnancy and child bearing; demonstrate knowledge of human development; demonstrate research appreciation, professional accountability, awareness of social and political factors related to health care, the requirements of relevant legislation; recognize and uphold the rights of patients and clients; develop helpful, caring and therapeutic relationships with patients, clients, families or friends using interpersonal and communication skills; identify learning needs of patients, clients, families or friends and participate in health promotion; demonstrate awareness of multidisciplinary roles and functioning; assign work to and supervise helpers; identify physical, psychological, social and spiritual needs of patients or clients within the plan of care and using a problem-solving approach; enable patients or clients to progress from dependence to independence or a peaceful death.

The long list of descriptive characteristics contained no detail of content. The knowledge and skill component of competence, the level and standard to be reached, the method of teaching, and the attainment and measurement of competence, were neither defined nor specified. The UKCC expected that competence would increase with experience and responsibility. It also emphasized caring as important, and argued that 'art' needed to be learnt alongside 'science'. Psychosocial content and health promotion were emphasized in the curriculum. Broad categories arising from the liberal arts replaced the 'medical model' and there was no mention of the nurse learning any specific practical clinical nursing skills. In fact, what was described were very general *aims* or hoped-for *outcomes* rather than precise competencies themselves.

This list of competencies was expected to replace the standing competencies listed in 1983 (UKCC, 1986a: 41, para 5.23). This duly occurred in the Statutory Instrument of 1989 (Statutory Instruments, 1989: No. 1456: 3930 rule 18A). The proposals of the UKCC (1986a), that a common foundation would underpin branch programmes, replaced the previous Training Rules. This Statutory Instrument made under the 1979 Act, Nurses, Midwives and Health Visitors: The Nurses, Midwives and Health Visitors (Registered Fever Nurses Amendment Rules and Training Amendment Rules) Approval Order 1989 amended the competencies in line with the Project 2000 publication:

(2) The Common Foundation Programme and Branch Programmes shall be designed to prepare the nursing student to assume the responsibilities and accountability that registration confers, and to prepare the nursing student to apply knowledge and skills to meet the nursing needs of individuals and of groups in health and in sickness in the area of practice of the Branch Programme and shall include enabling the student to achieve the following outcomes:–

(a) the identification of the social and health implications of pregnancy and childbearing, physical and mental handicap, disease, disability, or ageing for the individual, her or his friends, family and community;

(b) the recognition of common factors which contribute to, and those which adversely affect, physical, mental and social well-being of patients and clients and take appropriate action;

(c) the use of relevant literature and research to inform the practice of nursing;

(d) the appreciation of the influence of social, political and cultural factors in relation to health care;

(e) an understanding of the requirements of legislation relevant to the practice of nursing;

(f) the use of appropriate communication skills to enable the development of helpful caring relationships with patients and clients and their families and friends, and to initiate and conduct therapeutic relationships with patients and clients;

(g) the identification of health related learning needs of patients and clients, families and friends and to participate in health promotion;

(h) an understanding of the ethics of health care and of the nursing profession and the responsibilities which these impose on the nurse's professional practice;

(i) the identification of the needs of patients and clients to enable them to progress from varying degrees of dependence to maximum independence, or to a peaceful death;

(j) the identification of physical, psychological, social and spiritual needs of the patient or client; an awareness of values and concepts of individual care; the ability to devise a plan of care, contribute to its implementation and evaluation; and the demonstration of the application of the principles of a problem-solving approach to the practice of nursing;

(k) the ability to function effectively in a team and participate in a multi-professional approach to the care of patients and clients;

(l) the use of the appropriate channel of referral for matters not within her sphere of competence;

(m) the assignment of appropriate duties to others and the supervision, teaching and monitoring of assigned duties.

The quest for educational reform: inadequate reasons for change

The three reports were similar in their recommendations and aspirations for a move away from apprenticeship into forms of higher education with a broad liberal arts course to foster self-development. The impetus for urgent change seems to have been fuelled by very general feelings of discomfort and malaise amongst some nursing leaders. Concerns over recruitment and wastage were mentioned in all three reports. The RCN Commission was worried about recruitment and wastage but admitted that it was difficult to obtain accurate figures (RCN, 1985: 28, para. 3.10). The English National Board believed there was a 'crisis' situation, but in mental handicap nursing and mental nursing rather than general nursing. The UKCC thought that any problems with recruitment and retention did not provide an adequate argument for change. In reality, recruitment and wastage were even, in some senses, less of a problem in the 1980s than in previous decades.

Nevertheless it seems to have been assumed that by changing nurse preparation in the proposed ways recruitment and wastage among nurses would be improved. Yet, the National Audit Office found that overall wastage remained at 5 per cent from 1986, before the implementation of Project 2000, up to 1992, four years after the implementation (National Audit Office, 1992: 24, para. 4.29, table 4). The recruitment situation did not, however, improve, as time was to show.

Reactions to proposed changes: concerns about the practical basis of nursing

According to Jacka and Lewin (1987), the educationalist bias of the RCN Commission took for granted that apprenticeship was anachronistic and anti-educational: 'they do not bother with the possibility that there may be benign aspects: its influence is pervasive and baleful, compelling trainees to "march to the drumbeat of service"' (Jacka and Lewin, 1987: 32). Prussian drill, blind obedience and routine were contrasted with the melody and dance of student life, young people committed to learning, to personal and intellectual growth.

Although Jacka and Lewin regard this as an impasse, a result of a conflict of perceptions about nurse training, they did not disagree with the view that apprenticeship, as an organizational arrangement, assigned a low priority to education, or that it contained both stultifying and exploiting elements: the past hundred years had produced plenty of evidence to support this view. Nevertheless, they suggested that the principle of learning by example, by associating with a 'master', was sound. Explicit instruction played a smaller part in learning, especially craft learning, than many thought; and apprenticeship, even for some highly intellectual arts and crafts, was often the only way to transform a novice into an adept. Interpretation and qualification might narrow the gap, but the gap remained.

Jacka and Lewin believed that evidence needed to be sought to test whether the 'march to the drumbeat of service', the manpower demands of the hospital and the need for workers to give patient care, actually did constrain or hinder educational development of trainees. Evidence was also needed to ascertain the extent to which student nurses learnt by example, being close to the expert in action and watching his or her performance, during the three-year training.

Jacka and Lewin used two examples of practical nursing learning to illustrate their arguments. The first is the giving of an intramuscular injection; the second is the care of the dying. In the first example, the student nurse was taught in the classroom the relevant knowledge of anatomy, physiology and pharmacology. There she also learned the rudiments of an effective delivery of the drug; for example, the dart-thrower aimed at the orange. She learned tips on safety – locating within the upper outer quadrant of the buttock, and testing to make sure a vein has not been penetrated. Then she watched the performance of an expert: 'observing on a real live patient that combination of manual dexterity with the instrument, and the social finesse and aura of confidence which facilitate cooperation and relaxation' (Jacka and Lewin, 1987: 31). Professional craft knowledge, such as that used in motor maintenance, was mediated through the self-healing nature of the body and that element of care, the nurse–patient relationship, which existed because of the nature of human beings as social and moral agents.

Similarly, in caring for the dying patient, the nurse needed knowledge and skill of the disease process and the palliation of symptoms. Beyond this she needed the ability to build a relationship with someone who may be terrified, struggling to come to terms with the end of life. She needed to know how to respond, how to listen, how to see the patient as a whole person; what counted was not the quantity of time spent with the patient, but the quality of association. These capabilities were not acquired in the class-room, and not at all from psychology textbooks, rather, the nurse would learn by being with older experienced nurses who themselves possess these capacities and by watching them as they encounter these situations.

Just as nursing was abandoning this apprenticeship method of learning, others were arguing that the apprenticeship model should be emulated by other professions. The philosopher and educationalist, Mary Warnock, suggested that teachers should learn from nurses about a much stronger practice-based training. In the 1985 Richard Dimbleby Lecture, Warnock argued for a radical reform of teacher training which was too much part of higher education (Warnock, 1985). This she expanded three years later (Warnock, 1988).

Despite their recommendations, educationalists who proposed to remove the apprenticeship were also well aware that the practical base for nursing education was endangered by the proposed changes, and they sought to reaffirm it:

> It is unambiguously true that nurses need to do a great deal of their learning and to develop their skills in a clinical setting whether that setting is the hospital or, as it must increasingly be, the community. Any proposals which depart from this axiom deserve to be rejected out of hand.
>
> (RCN, 1985: 7–8, para.1.3)

Harry Judge himself was keen to emphasize that theory and practice could have a 'fruitful relationship'. As he stated in an interview: 'My perspective is not one which stresses the theoretical or the academic over and against the practical' (Fleming, 1985: 54). Despite such affirmations, concerns continued that the move into higher education would result in a more theoretical and less practical approach to preparing nurses. This was clear from the UKCC consultations and the responses.

Celia Davies, the Project Officer, appears to have had a deep influence on the impetus and direction of changing nursing. She provides some insight on this influence and her own motivations in a retrospective, published in 1995. As she toured the country in 1984–85, outlining to a wide variety of groups the aims of the UKCC nurse education project, Davies interpreted reactions as demonstrating that nurses did not want mere reform of education but 'root and branch reform of the nature and conditions of nursing itself' (Davies, 1995: 3). She quoted the statement from the RCN Commission (1985), repeated by the UKCC (1986a), that nurse education during this period was reminiscent of a 19th century teachers' training college. And, referring to a study by Lesley Mackay (1989), which had interviewed nurses, Davies argued that nurses were discontented. But this evidence was selectively used by Davies. The other finding of Mackay, which Davies omitted, was that nurses had a strong sense of vocation and gained satisfaction from the care they gave.

By 1995, dissatisfaction and lack of commitment amongst nurses appears to have been acknowledged, evidenced by the tendency for nurses to seek to collect paper certificates and move from job to job. Davies seems to have felt the need to defend the new system against this criticism, arguing that this was no different to the dissatisfaction and lack of commitment of the 1960s. Then Menzies (1960) found that senior nurses changed jobs frequently and 'were unusually prone to seek postgraduate training' (Davies, 1995: 97). But evidence from that period of the 1960s (for example, Dutton, 1968) shows that the opposite was true. Indeed, Menzies' small-scale study did not provide reliable evidence to support Davies's case. Although Davies referred to Project Paper 7 (UKCC, 1986b), and admitted that not everyone 'was convinced about the whole package of proposals and there was some serious questioning of aspects of the report', she neverthe-less believed that the overall tenor of the profession's response was welcoming (Davies, 1995: 112). She omitted any details of what was, by her own admission, 'serious questioning'. Arguably, she underplayed criticisms of proposed changes from within the grass-roots of the profession, although she did admit on the record that the medical profession, who were not represented on the UKCC Committee, were unhappy with the proposed changes. By the year 2000, Davies would express serious concerns about nursing developments, as Chapter 6 will show.

The medical responses

Doctors were indeed concerned about the proposed changes to nursing. The Central Committee for Hospital Medical Services (CCHMS) was reported by the *British Medical Journal* (*BMJ*, 1986: 1585–86) as being worried by the Project 2000 proposals. Although members were concerned not to be accused of being 'fuddy duddies', they were critical that no nurse currently employed in clinical duties was on the UKCC committee. The document had instead been prepared by 13 nurse educators, four academ-ics in the theory of education, and two senior nurse administrators.

Mary White thought the project was a disaster for nursing: 'Nursing was essentially a practical skill and was best learnt as an apprentice not in a technical college'. John Dewar hoped ward sisters and staff nurses who were critical of the proposals would make their views known directly rather than through managers. He was concerned about the reduced training capacity.

W. J. Appleyard was worried at the radical nature of the proposals and thought that, if implemented, they would alter the whole pattern of care in hospitals. Anne Grüneberg was more positive about the proposals, seeing the need to change the existing system. But J. M. Cundy believed the idea of nursing aides should be rejected. L. P. Harvey thought the numbers of nurses that were expected to be recruited was unrealistic, while Nuala Sterling thought some parts of the document should be accepted.

Brendan Devlin, Consultant Surgeon at North Tees General Hospital, Stockton, Cleveland, writing in *Nursing Times* (Devlin, 1987: 29–30), expressed his deep concerns about the proposals. The medical response to the Project 2000 proposals was muted, but doctors were not consulted. The UKCC had not only failed to involve doctors, but it had also had no practical clinical nurse among its members. He argued that the reforms would separate nurse education from clinical practice and that nursing did not need people who collected advanced academic qualifications. He believed that student nurses should train on the wards and that enrolled nurses should be retained. He also thought that drop-out figures were unconvincing in that nursing was no different to other professions in the drop-out rates. In fact he thought that the transfer of nurse education further away from the patient was likely to increase the rate. The movement of education out of the NHS was also likely to politicize decision-making: 'A purely academic environment will isolate the trainees and the trainers from the real world of clinical practice so let's keep the student nurses where the action is.'

Brian Gibberd (1988: 182–183), Consultant Physician at Westminster Hospital, London, echoed many of these same concerns. Recruitment would not be improved, neither would wastage be reduced, by changing the educational methods. The person who was practising the profession was often better at educating students than the educationalist, who was not a teacher. As it was, the UK nursing profession was held in high regard by other countries. Any problems would not be remedied by Project 2000, and hence, Gibberd thought, other options apart from Project 2000 needed to be considered. Nurses should be welcomed for their practical skills and not just academic achievement: 'The UKCC seems to regard nursing as a profession that needs to compete with universities and business on an academic basis, rather than as a profession that concentrates on patient care.'

Governmental responses

Was the government persuaded then by the call from the sociologists and educationalists who sought radical change? For one prospective Member of Parliament, Gillian Shepherd (*sic*) (Dickson, 1987: 28), (presumably Gillian Shepherd, later a member of the Conservative cabinet, and a

Secretary of State for Education), the arguments were persuasive. Indeed, she thought that nursing was merely following teacher training in its call for a college-based education. She dismissed the argument that under Project 2000 student nurses would become too academic and theoretical. But, as Warnock had already warned, teacher training would be recognized increasingly as problematic over the next decade.

John Moore, the Minister for Health, appeared also to be concerned that nurse training would become less practical if Project 2000 was adopted. In 1988, he wrote to Audrey Emerton, Chairman of the UKCC, that he agreed to introduce Project 2000, *on the condition that* assurance be given that the clinical base for nurse education would not be lost:

> You will be aware that consultations revealed considerable misunderstanding of the Council's intentions, and fears that the changes would place nurse education predominantly in a classroom setting thus unacceptably reducing the practical, patient-orientated content of training. It is therefore important to place on record our joint understanding that nursing education must retain its clinical focus, and that students will not spend substantially less time in clinical areas than at present. The difference is that their contribution to patient care will be better aligned to the level of theoretical grounding and practical experience which they have attained.
>
> (Moore, 1988)

Moore seemed to be assuming that the new model of nurse education he was agreeing to was a continuation of the apprenticeship model but underpinned by a more theoretical knowledge base. He appeared to believe that the clinical focus of nurse preparation would be unchanged. Student nurses had been similarly concerned but their concerns, unlike the Minister's, were summarily dismissed in the UKCC Project Paper 7.

Behind the introduction of Project 2000 was an ideological battle. In Davies's view (1995), nursing was an expression of the gendered division in society. This was how she interpreted her own battles to have Project 2000 implemented. Her role was to bring this view, that nursing exemplified conflict, division and struggle, into the consciousness of nurses and those who formed opinions and policy in the profession. Tony Delamothe, Assistant Editor of the *British Medical Journal*, writing in a series of articles in the *BMJ* (Delamothe, 1988a, b, c, d, e, f) shared Davies's view. Delamothe (1988g: 1344) argued that nursing was no longer a vocation for the majority of nurses: 'Few nurses now regard what they do as a vocation; most come into nursing expecting a career, comparable with other careers.' Mackay's work in 1989, however, questioned this statement. So did another study published that same year by Nessling (1989), which specifically found nurses' motivations to be primarily vocational rather than careerist.

Whether the government appreciated the revolutionary nature of change being proposed by sociologists and educationalists on nursing policy-making committees in the mid-1980s is questionable. According to Davies (1995: 118) the UKCC was keen to influence the government by highlighting 'the demographic threat', by arguing that falling birth rates meant that nursing could not recruit such high numbers from the age group of 18-year-old women, so that the status quo was not an option. Perhaps the government thought it was approving merely a change of venue for nurse education, but it was actually approving a change of content that was ideologically driven.

A new kind of nurse and a new form of nursing

By radically redefining training into a more general education, the nursing bodies were in fact, intentionally or unintentionally, redefining the role of the registered nurse. This may well be the quintessential issue. The changes to nurse education were not merely to produce 'educated' nurses, doing the same job as before, but with more time and less pressure for their training, but a different breed of nurse, whose role would not necessarily be primarily that of addressing the patient's personal practical needs.

This insight corresponds with the RCN *Comments on the UKCC's Project 2000 Proposals* (1986), which referred to a statement by Harry Judge that nursing could now make itself whatever it wanted to be, providing it could state its wants clearly and unambiguously. The RCN's comment was *not* that the government would ensure that nursing was responsive to patient service first and foremost, but that the future of nursing was in the hands of no one else but the 'profession', that is, its élite bureaucracy, not its members. And the next section of the comment proceeds to discuss the new concepts – put forward by the UKCC – of the registered practitioner and the specialist practitioner.

It seems that the government in 1988 itself acknowledged some change in the nature of nursing, for it advocated and affirmed the importance of a new support worker role. The Secretary of State for Social Services agreed to the introduction of Project 2000 and the change in nurse education provided it took place alongside the development of a new support worker. As John Moore wrote in his letter to Audrey Emerton:

> . . . we also place great weight on the proposals being worked up for a new range of support workers to be deployed under the direction of the profes- sional nurse, with appropriate opportunities for such support workers to progress to nurse education and training if they have the desire and capacity to do so. There have been important developments since the

Project 2000 proposals were submitted which will have a bearing on the support worker proposals, notably the work of the National Council for Vocational Qualifications and the creation of a training consortium for the care sector. A start has been made in defining and developing the role and training of support workers for professional staff building on the work done for the YTS Feasibility Study.

(Moore, 1988)

The government seems to have envisaged that the practical bulk of nursing care when no longer performed by student nurses as part of their apprenticeship training would be taken over by health care assistants, and not by qualified and registered nurses. The UKCC (1986) had itself advocated some kind of nursing assistant or 'aide' to boost the manpower requirements.

While welcoming the new kind of nurse to be ushered in by Project 2000, some nursing writers also highlighted a worry about the proposed increased use of untrained nursing assistants. Turner and Dickson (1988: 12–13), for example, in an article in the *Nursing Times* headed 'Project 2000: a new dawn for nursing?', noted that the acceptance of Project 2000 by the government 'opened the way for a radically new type of nurse' to take nursing into the next century. Nevertheless they suggested that questions were being asked as to whether a 'horde of unqualified helpers' would lower standards, and indeed, whether widening the entry gate for such helpers contradicted the idea of fostering closer links with higher education in order to create a more autonomous practitioner. It appears that John Moore envisaged a smaller workforce of trained professional nurses, an élite, supervising 'an army of helpers, many of them only minimally trained' (Salvage, 1988: 1553).

Conclusion

Despite arguments to the contrary, both from within the profession and outside, by 1985 and 1986 nursing's professional bodies had begun the shift of nurse education away from hierarchy, prescriptions, rules and examinations into a collegiate, self-reliant, flexible and self-directed method of learning. Individual nurses were to assume responsibility for their own educational standards and development. They were to be responsible for acquiring competencies, broadly defined as applied knowledge, skill and attitudes. These competencies would not be linked to a 'medical model' but to a 'nursing model'. The practice component of training would be supernumerary, according to the student's needs rather than service needs. The kind of knowledge that the qualified nurse of the future needed would depend on what she was expected to do. It appeared

that the nursing role itself would be subject to change. To a great extent
this was not merely a practical issue but a philosophical and ideological
one.

CHAPTER 3

Educating for competence? Nurse education 1985–1999

Introduction

The previous chapters have charted the way that, in the wake of the Briggs Report, the apprenticeship model of nurse training was completely discarded and the legislative framework was set up entrusting the development of a new model of nursing into the hands of the professional bodies, the UKCC and, in England, the ENB. These bodies sought to define nurse education and to set out in very general terms the content of the curriculum. But problems surfaced over the lack of a definition of competence. The key question arises, therefore, as to how nurses were prepared to be competent. A full account of the reviews, official and unofficial, is given in this chapter with a view to providing evidence about how the new educational system was shaping nurses to be competent and fit for practice. The largest body of evidence comes from England, but where other evidence exists it is also considered. This Chapter expands and develops an earlier analysis (Bradshaw, 1997, 1998).

Preparation for nursing competence

The responsibility of the professional bodies: regulating nursing education

The implementation of Project 2000 courses began gradually from September 1989. Project 2000 was underpinned by a new self-regulatory framework. Fundamental to the newly devised codes of conduct of the reconstituted nursing, midwifery and health visiting professions were the two pillars upon which they now rested, the *autonomy* and *accountability* of the individual registered practitioner. This was enshrined by the UKCC in its regulatory publications sent to all registered practitioners (UKCC, 1984, 1989a, 1992a, 1992b, 1996a). Each registered practitioner was now legally responsible and personally accountable for her own actions. No one else could answer for the practitioner and it was no defence for the practitioner to say that she was acting on someone else's orders. She needed to maintain and improve her competence, acknowledge limitations in that competence, ensure that not only her acts, but also her omissions, that lay within her sphere of responsibility, were not detrimental to the interests, condition or safety of her patients. She had to acknowledge any limitations in her knowledge and competence, and decline to perform duties unless able to perform them in a safe and skilled manner.

Much of the new philosophy, which was to underpin nursing education both pre- and post-registration, imagined that the conventional career of nursing had now collapsed. Skills were to be transferable as registered nurses moved in a variety of career paths. This philosophy was espoused by Celia Davies in her 1990 paper 'The Collapse of the Conventional Career', written for the ENB (Davies, 1990). Drawing on the management theory of Charles Handy (1984, 1989), Davies argued that patterns of work were changing, and suggested that 'flexible specialization' was the key to understanding the 'business' culture of health care in which nursing operated and needed to fit (1990: 1, 13). This concept, which distanced the nurse from the moral basis of her calling, locating her career in the utilitarian market place, was to have a fundamental effect on nurse preparation. Handy, interestingly, was later to admit the ethical weakness of this ideology (Handy, 1998).

A lack of definition for competence required of the nursing role

The national syllabus had ended, and a new curriculum developed which would allow educational institutions freedom to individualize it. The educational philosophy developed in the 1980s by Davies amongst others was enshrined in the ENB *Regulations and Guidelines for the Approval of Institutions and Courses* (1993a). Standards and competencies were referred to as the basis of the nurse's responsibility and accountability, but they were not defined. The document did not specify the content of any courses. Course content should be determined by the individual student's professional needs and curriculum design should be flexible. Different colleges were likely to have differing content in their courses. As to learning outcomes, the document stated that 'learning outcomes must be identified within units of learning; *broad parameters only should be given*' (ENB, 1993a: 1.15, para. 7.3; my italics).

Guidelines were deliberately vague. So, for example, the document stated that in areas of practical placement where students were supervised:

Staff should demonstrate enthusiasm to share their expertise, develop professional competencies and extend the boundaries of knowledge. The qualified staff should, where appropriate, hold the specialist qualification which is relevant to the particular care area.

(ENB, 1993a: 2.17, para. 7.4.5.g)

Prescriptive regulations were confined to the number of practical hours needed to be worked. Definitions, apparently circular, directed that students should learn *how* to learn. Educational 'process' assumed dominance. Training 'outcomes', the learning of detailed and specified skills and procedures, were displaced. As prefigured earlier in educational change, 'chalk and talk' and 'rote learning' were ended, and replaced by a more fluid and creative self-directed method of 'development'.

Updated documents continued to reflect a similar approach. Curriculum development was 'to produce a "knowledgeable doer" capable of competent and research aware practice'. Benchmarks for excellence were to be found in the 10 Key Characteristics of expert practice contained in a 1991 ENB Publication (ENB, 1994: 4). These characteristics (ENB, 1991) broadly reflected the legislation detailed in Statutory Instruments of 1983 and 1989.

In the main, this new document built on existing course content (UKCC, 1988, 1989b). The Common Foundation Programme reiterated a similar 'indicative' content which was vague and unspecified, but focused on the theoretical, conceptual, psychosocial, managerial and political knowledge of the nurse. Five categories were covered: nursing; the development of the individual, human growth and development; definitions of health, wellness, illness, care and cure; health care systems; and socialization and education. Only one category, out of 38 listed in the course of the five headings, was concerned with disease and pathological process and included the nature and causation of disease, aspects of microbiology and pharmacology and their application to the provision of care. But it was also specified that this should include supportive (complementary) therapies (ENB, 1994: 9–10).

Statements on the Branch Programme in Adult Nursing allowed for wide interpretation and did not mention anything concrete that would be measurable or testable. Nursing skills, mentioned in the 'indicative content' remained broad and undefined: 'adaptation of essential (core) nursing skills associated with activities of daily living required to promote individual patient's maximum health potential and independence'; and 'complex nursing skills required in the management of medical and surgical emergencies and accidents and specialized technological procedures unique to adult nursing'. Significantly, the programme had no

mention of the disease process at all, neither was there mention of microbiology, pharmacology, or indeed, anatomy and physiology. Instead, the
first statement focused the remaining content: 'health promotion and
prevention of ill health as they relate to the healthy, episodically acute and
longer term ill individual across the age spectrum and the meeting of
health care targets' (ENB, 1994: 13).

That nurses should receive an education was an aim rather than an
outcome measure of what this education would enable the nurse to do for
patients. There were no details of procedures, tasks or ways of achievement. Instead nursing theories and philosophies of self-reflection
dominated the curriculum (Bradshaw, 1995). Education was one remove
from any answer to the question 'How do I give an injection?', for
example. This was because 'education' was not 'training'. The purpose of
education was personal and intellectual development, as opposed to the
purpose of training, which was related to performance.

The repercussions caused by the lack of set standards and procedures
for registration had implications for what might be counted as specialist
post-registration. The ENB *Guidelines for Programmes Leading to the
Qualification of Specialist Practitioner* enumerated ten key characteristics
of the expert practitioner: accountability; clinical skills; use of research;
team work; innovation; health promotion; staff development; resource
management; quality of care; and management of change (ENB, 1995: 2).

The only specialist areas listed were those in the community: general
practice nursing; community mental health nursing; community mental
handicap/learning disability nursing; community children's nursing;
public health nursing – health visiting; occupational health nursing;
community nursing in the home – district nursing; and school nursing.
Guidelines for curriculum design and development were expected to be
flexible, modular, linked to a higher education accreditation system, and
to allow credit for prior learning and prior experiential learning.

The UKCC *Standards for Education and Practice Following
Registration* (1994a) were appended to the ENB document. The
standards in this document, upon which the ENB guidelines were based,
were broad principles to be applied by institutions in different ways 'to
offer meaningful, adaptable and appropriate courses of education' (ENB,
1995: 23, Annexe 1, para. 16). Standards of specialist practice were not
differentiated from those of registration. In all areas nurses were expected
to assess, plan, implement and evaluate care, empower patients and
clients, take responsibility, and often, counsel patients.

Where specific skills were mentioned, as for example with regard to
'diagnostic, therapeutic, resuscitative and technological procedures and
techniques' (ENB, 1995: 24, Annexe 2, para. 19.5), specific knowledge and

skill components were not defined, and no measurable level of skill was specified. No distinction was drawn between what constituted the 'ordinary level' of knowledge and skill expected of every registered nurse, and the level of knowledge and skill expected at an 'advanced level' from the specialist nurse.

Hence, under the heading, 'Standards for Specialist Community Nursing Education and Practice' (ENB, 1995: 24, Annexe 3, para. 20), the document stated that the nurse should achieve the following common core outcomes derived as appropriate from a specific area of specialist nursing practice, one of which was to prescribe from a nursing formulary where the legislation permitted. Requisite knowledge and skill needed for the nurse to take on such a role was not specified.

In February 1996 the new *Regulations and Guidelines for the Approval of Institutions and Programmes* was produced (ENB, 1996). The intention was to review the document annually, with a major review to be undertaken 1996/1997. As the document stated:

> This revised set of pages for the Regulations and Guidelines Folder does not contain any major policy changes. However, some of the wording in the document has been altered to make it more user friendly and to avoid duplication.
>
> (ENB, 1996: iv)

Attention was drawn to the distinction in the document between the use of the words 'must' or 'will' to denote regulations, and 'should' or 'may' to denote guidelines (ENB, 1996: iv). The document remained flexible, and non-prescriptive, generally focusing on broad issues but leaving details to the institution to interpret in its own way.

Hence, for example, under 'Assessment Strategy' the document stated that a portfolio of learning must be compiled and maintained by each student. The purpose of this was to provide cumulative information about the student's achievement and progress, demonstrating the interrelationship of theory and practice. Cause for concern relating to progress must be entered in the portfolio and recorded in the assessment documentation (ENB, 1996: 5.11, paras. 2.1.2–2.1.4).

Guidelines only were given about the content of the portfolio, which might include the student's record of initiatives demonstrating analytical and problem-solving skills, learning contracts and outcomes of these, reference to relevant reading and the application of research findings, and the student's achievement of outcomes and learning through reflection (ENB, 1996: 5.11, para. 2.1.5). No concrete or objective content or measures of that content were suggested or specified.

Similarly vague was the reference to supervision of clinical practice. Assessment of practice should include the collection of a range of information to serve as a basis for student/assessor discussion about knowledge, skills, attitudes and understanding. The assessor must directly observe the student's performance in the practice setting and should consult relevant colleagues about the student's progress. The outcome of assessment and action agreed must be documented (ENB, 1996: 5.13, paras. 2.3.6–2.3.9). No criteria of what constituted performance and progress were given. No measures for what the assessor was assessing were stated.

From regulations to standards but no real change

In 1997 the *Regulations and Guidelines for the Approval of Institutions and Courses* was replaced by *Standards for Approval of Higher Education Institutions and Programmes* (1997a). Significantly, in the Foreword, the Chairman, Ron De Witt, and the Chief Executive, Anthony Smith, felt the need to state that the change from 'regulations and guidelines to standards and criteria' was not 'merely cosmetic but a fundamental re-clarification and re-affirmation of those structures, processes and outcomes which are deemed to result in quality professional education for quality care' (ENB, 1997a: 2). Hence, there was no real change in the ENB regulations from 1993 to 1997.

Not only was the concept of 'competence' not mentioned, but what this statement declared was that there had indeed been no fundamental change. The document was intended only to re-clarify and re-affirm what was being replaced. In other words it was the language and structure of the document which was different. This might indicate a concern to describe 'standards', but no specific standards were set. Indeed, the Foreword stated that the Board was 'confident that the new standards are appropriate, comprehensive and measurable' but no measures were defined.

Hence, although the document used terms such as 'standards' and 'quality', there were no clear mechanisms, objective tests, or specific measures imposed on the institutions. This is ironic, given that the introduction to the document stated: 'As a result of the national consultations undertaken, the Board believes that the standards are grounded in reality and are achievable and measurable' (ENB, 1997a: 3). There was nothing new required of the higher education institutions wishing to train nurses: 'The Board wishes to emphasize that the standards contain no essentially new requirements of the higher education institutions. The current expectations have been made explicit' (ENB, 1997a: 3). What had changed, then, was only the format. It was a cosmetic change.

The bulk of the document contained the 18 standards designed to create the ten key characteristics for continuing professional education (ENB, 1991). These were to enable nurses, midwives and health visitors to be: innovative in their practice; responsive to changing demand; resourceful in their methods of working; able to work as change agents; able to share good practice and knowledge; adaptable to changing health care needs; challenging and creative in their practice; self-reliant in their way of working; and accountable for their work (ENB, 1997a: 5).

These standards were: the higher education institution as an organization; meeting workforce requirements; strategic and operational management of nursing/midwifery/ health visiting education; staff resource, staff development; research and development; physical and learning resources; practice experience; lecturer's involvement in nursing/midwifery/health visiting practice; student admissions; curriculum design and development; curriculum and assessment; assessment process; assessors of practice; external examiners; student support; programme management; fitness for purpose, practice and award.

Standards were underpinned by criteria which tended to be vague statements that contained few details and were therefore open to extremely wide interpretation. For example, Standard 2, 'Meeting workforce requirements', had two criteria – first:

> Collaboration, partnership and professional alliances support practice-focused education reflecting national and local workforce trends and priorities.

and second:

> Mechanisms are in place to ensure that workforce demands are met.
> (ENB, 1997a: 18–19)

Standard 8, 'Practice experience', had ten criteria, in which the eighth stated:

> A named person who holds effective first level registration on the Professional Register and other professional and academic qualifications and experience commensurate with the context of care delivery supervises and assesses students in health care settings.
> (ENB, 1997a: 22–23)

Whether this supervisor was assessed as competent, how he or she was tested as such, was not set out by this circular definition.

Standard 11, 'Curriculum design and development', stated:

> Curriculum design and development reflect contemporary educational approaches and health care practice.

The 12 criteria included such topics as:

> The staff resource is clearly identified in relation to the programme.

> Curriculum is founded on professional and academic knowledge, practice and education which are evidence/research-based where possible.

> The curriculum provides the opportunity to equip practitioners to deliver care in a multi-cultural context and to challenge discriminatory practices.
>
> (ENB, 1997a: 24)

And Standard 12 'Curriculum and assessment', included among the assessment strategy criteria:

> contains descriptors which discriminate how the acquisition of knowledge, skills and attitudes is applied and assessed at different academic and professional levels;

and also:

> requires the student to demonstrate competence within practice through the achievement of learning outcomes in both theory and practice.
>
> (ENB, 1997a: 25)

Assessment methods were not prescribed.

What is striking in this document, and is also reflected in the *Guidelines for External Examiners* (ENB, 1997b) is how little relevance it seems to bear to the specific function of nursing, midwifery or health visiting: what the professional should be able to *do*. Indeed, it could be used as a document for any course of study loosely designed as a preparation for the workplace. It may be concluded that, despite the variety of UKCC and ENB statements on quality and standards, nurse education was now supported by a philosophy that placed responsibility on the individual practitioner to define and assess her own standard of competency. Although statements suggested that educational standards were measurable, neither standards nor measures were defined or prescribed. Three questions remained. What was the standard of competency the nurse needed to attain to be fit for her job? How was the nurse prepared to reach this standard? What measures were used to evaluate attainment, that is, that the goal has been reached satisfactorily? Some insight into ENB thinking on this term 'measure' is afforded by its guidelines for educational audit.

Fitness for what purpose?

The ENB guidelines on educational audit presupposed nursing education to be a journey rather than a destination (Jean Hooper, Chairman, ENB, 1993b: 4). They were not intended to be prescriptive or restrictive but to develop quality mechanisms. Each institution was seen as unique and would thus offer a different education. There was to be no 'blueprint' for nursing education. Neither was there to be a blueprint for quality. Quality in nursing education was seen as relative according to the fitness for purpose, which was viewed as central, but this fitness for purpose was not defined. Quality, a 'cultural process', reflected the values and views of the participants and was related to 'educational effectiveness' (ENB, 1993b: 7). Five factors identified as factors for quality assessment were: goal achievement; resource acquisition; internal processes; participant satisfaction; and social justice (ENB, 1993b: 11).

Effectiveness of learning experiences could be evaluated by, for example, student evaluation data, student achievement of clinical competencies, and relevance of placement to curriculum objectives identified in documentation. Whether the clinical experience enabled the student to achieve her competencies might be ascertained through, for example, continuous clinical assessment, board of examiners' reports and external examiners' reports. Evidence of formal preparation of placement staff or mentors might be, for example, by the number of first-level staff holding 997/998 teaching certificates, degrees or in-service education courses (ENB, 1993b: 68–71). Despite long lists such as these, no concrete and objective measures of assessment of competencies for nursing students, theoretical or practical, were suggested or intended.

Indeed, the ENB courses 997 and 998, used to prepare teachers and assessors, as Nicklin and Kenworthy (1995) stated, were themselves based on an experiential framework which did not seek to measure learning outcomes because it was considered that they measured only a narrow band of cognitive skills. The strategy for educating nurse educators was the same as that for educating adult students: an adult-learning model which relied on self-direction and individual experience rather than what Nicklin and Kenworthy (1995: 27) called 'rationality-based' models of learning. Yet this model of education, as Nicklin and Kenworthy (1995: 27) stated in two sentences that were not expanded or explored, was not without criticism: 'Needless to say many of these assumptions have been vigorously challenged. This model has however been very influential in recent years.'

The student progressed through levels of learning through placements by 'exposure to experience', eventually 'internalizing' and 'disseminating' the experience. The outcomes were 'behaviours' assessed as 'the ability to solve problems, analyse and interpret situations and data' as well as abilities of advocacy, counselling, and the formation of judgmental skills. The final point, 'dissemination', was demonstrated by self-assessment, peer assessment and the desire to set objectives for continuing development (Nicklin and Kenworthy, 1995: 65–66). Educational effectiveness for nursing practice was clearly seen as a relative concept without intrinsic content, a fluid and movable process. Most importantly, the role and function for which the student was to be prepared, that is, the nursing purpose and destination, was left blurred and undefined.

Evaluation of pre-registration nursing education

Defining and assessing 'competence' in nurse education

Already, in 1992, the National Audit Office report, *Nursing Education: Implementation of Project 2000 in England*, had found concern among managers about nurses' practical skills. Although they thought that student nurses were better able to ask searching questions as a result of their wider education, all levels of management expressed concerns that on qualification Project 2000 nurses' practical skills would be less well developed than those of the traditional nurse. They doubted whether this new type of nurse would be able to contribute as much to the ward team (National Audit Office, 1992: 26, para 4.40). This concern would be reinforced by evidence over the following years.

Problems for nursing teachers and students over defining competence

Because neither the UKCC nor the ENB defined 'competency' there was a problem for the registered nurse of knowing whether he or she was competent. Even an influential nursing leader admitted that competence was guesswork (Castledine, 1994: 103): 'The achievement and degree of expertise needed in carrying out a required competency is [also] not covered, leaving the practitioner to guess what level they should reach.'

A study by Bedford, Phillips, Robinson and Schostak (1993) highlighted the profound difficulties, among both nursing students and nursing teachers, in defining and assessing competence. The researchers suggested that definitions of competence and assessment within 'academic debate' and 'official texts' needed to be distinguished from the 'beliefs concerning competence that arise during the course of practice' (Bedford et al., 1993: 31).

The 'official texts' from the UKCC and ENB did not define competencies, other than very vaguely. Assessment of competency had become a subjective interpretation, with obvious inconsistencies and differences of opinion. As one student, interviewed for the study, was quoted: '. . . what I really found with the clinical objectives is that they're very ambiguous, they don't really give a level.' (Bedford et al., 1993: 66–67). This student had found in the example she gave, the taking of a temperature, that different assessors had different criteria for assessing her competency.

Yet, as the authors of the study wrote: 'It would seem that subjectivity and multiple interpretation are inevitable in assessment' (Bedford et al., 1993: 67). A fully standardized approach to assessing practice is 'counter educational'. The principles of classification differed in each case and unlike a behavioural model which seeks to classify and standardize behaviour, 'it will not be possible to assure homogeneity' (Bedford et al., 1993: 67).

The case referred to in the study, the checking of a temperature, is an unusual example of a competency. Many nurses interviewed, in line with UKCC and ENB philosophy described above, seemed to regard the acquisition of competencies as whatever made for problem-solving, communication and management. Competence was now 'multidimensional . . . a new form of competence. That it's not the skills based competence that we had before, it's much more open, learning, flexible, outcomes type of thing' (Bedford et al., 1993: 35). As Bedford et al. wrote: 'At its broadest, competence includes "life experience"' (Bedford et al., 1993: 36).

Skills for assessment of competence of the nurse, then, rejected the former, traditional assessment systems, formal examinations of both theory and practice, and instead adopted negotiated methods such as learning contracts, critical incident analysis, interviewing each other, situational analysis and reflection and dialogue-facilitating self-assessment, underpinned by the development of judgement (Bedford et al., 1993: 77–78). Although as to this last point, the authors also found that: 'There will always be some areas of disagreement where judgement is involved' (Bedford et al., 1993: 134).

The standard of nursing care was deliberately not defined: 'The product of the work of professionals is not amenable to the same kind of standardization as say production-line cars . . . Standardization is, in effect, the opposite to professional standards' (Bedford et al., 1993: 156).

Educational preparation lacking in practical skills, structure and standards

Research studies evaluating Project 2000 educational courses have focused on the experiences and opinions of nursing students, nurses and managers (Robinson, 1993; Elkan, Hillman and Robinson, 1993; Jowett, Walton and Payne, 1994; Macleod Clark, Maben and Jones, 1996). They did not seek to supply any objective evaluation of the suitability of courses to provide the nurse with a defined and measured knowledge, skill or ability that made her competent to practise. Even so, opinions pointed to problems.

Robinson's study stated: 'When asked about disadvantages of Project 2000 many practitioners felt that students are not provided with enough placement experience to develop adequate basic skills' (Robinson, 1993: 38). The study by Elkan et al. reported on the student-centred nature of learning, which meant that students defined and negotiated their own learning needs. They also found evidence that students wanted more structure and had reservations about self-directed learning methods. But they interpreted students' reservations about the fitness of their education to be the result of a lack of understanding or, indeed, resource limitations.

Elkan et al. (1993: 6–7) devoted two pages to the views of one student published in a nursing journal (Allen, 1990). Allen wrote that most nursing students saw themselves as frontline caregivers 'armed with the necessary task-orientated skills'; despite this, however 'such has been the focus on self and society, interpersonal skills, environmental health and sociologese, that sometimes I have to remind myself that we are not budding social scientists and that one day we will be nursing' (Allen, 1990: 43).

But Elkan et al. interpreted Allen's opinion as equivocal, and indeed, Allen seems to undergo a changed consciousness. By 1993 she was arguing that the movement from the 'hierarchical, task-oriented' model of training towards 'a more humanistic, student-centred approach' was welcome because it empowers nurses and hence empowers patients (Allen, 1993: 57). Students who complained about the fitness of their courses to prepare them as practical nurses are categorized in the study by Elkan et al. under the heading 'moaners' (1993: 56).

Jowett et al.'s study also noted the view that there was too much time and emphasis given to academic subjects such as sociology and psychology 'and too little to the crux areas of nursing' (Jowett et al., 1994: 123). The majority of Jowett's student interviewees 'felt that their level of achievement was satisfactory'; a sixth, however, felt inadequately prepared because of inappropriate placements. 'The widely held sense of achieve-ment was clear in the student who stated that "I am happy with my practical skills" . . .' (Jowett et al., 1994: 101). The question whether such self-assessment of attainment reflected objective standards of attainment and achievement, competence and safety, was not discussed. How did the student know what he or she did not know they did not know?

Project 2000 students in a study by While, Roberts and Fitzpatrick (1995) also emphasized the lack of practical experience: 'It was inter-esting that P2000 diploma programme participants identified nursing skills as an area of perceived confidence deficit . . .' (While et al., 1995: 220). According to While: 'There are all sorts of points students raised about Project 2000 which in the fullness of time will no doubt be remedied. The lack of practical experience was emphasized' (While, 1996: 51). Course content was variable and unspecified. One student was quoted as saying, 'They are really trying to get away from practical assessments on the ward, aseptic techniques and drug rounds. But I think it would have helped if they had been a bit more specific about the practical' (While, 1996: 51).

Macleod Clark et al. (1996) reached similar conclusion from their study into the perceptions of students, managers, teachers and practitioners regarding Project 2000. Too much theory was learnt at the expense of practical skills, although this defect was remedied in the months after registration. Educational philosophy underpinning nurse education had become that of health and health promotion rather than disease (Lask, Smith and Masterson, 1994). This approach marked a shift of emphasis in the content of nursing curricula from the biomedical towards the psychosocial and from the practical to the theoretical.

The major threat to the confidence of nursing students on placement was 'not being able to do "tasks" such as take temperatures, blood pressures, and catheter care' (Eraut, Alderton, Boylan and Wraight, 1995: 80). Emphasis on the ward was still placed on the tasks, on what the nurse could do, despite what was being taught theoretically. From observation Eraut et al. noted that students were awkward handling patients, in, for example, changing sheets. Indeed, they ignored such aspects of care, focusing on more dextrous technical tasks. Even then they breached the principles of cross-infection. Eraut et al. (1995) suggested that students were unused to activities which systematically studied the knowledge-base relevant to a particular case, curricula were uncoordinated, and too health-focused. They recommended that students should develop a repertoire of simple practical skills to enter placements with credibility. They also needed basic relevant biological knowledge, task and duty allocation related to their level of competence, and explicit training in learning from experience. Furthermore, there were few conceptual frameworks available for constructing overall programme plans and integrating relevant scientific knowledge with education and practice.

Eraut et al. (1995) saw their own work as supporting an earlier study by White, Riley, Davies and Twinn (1993). This study found a real concern, particularly among practitioners, about the abilities of Project 2000 students in both adult nursing and mental health branches upon qualification. In both branches there was also confusion among practitioners about the level of practice at which students were assessed at each stage, and assessment of student practice itself 'was undertaken with various levels of expertise and rigour' (White et al., 1993: 199–200).

White et al. suggested that in their placements in both branches students expressed apprehension about their comparatively low level of skill development, and a lack of knowledge about whether responsibility for this lay with themselves, the practitioners or their tutors. Assessment of student practice across both branches was problematic, and the instruments for so doing were ambiguous and open to considerable subjective variation:

> Indeed, practice was often judged independent of a practitioner having witnessed it, but rather on an articulation by the student of unobserved practice, or through discussion with others.
>
> (White et al., 1993: 206)

There was widespread uncertainty about the required educational level both among students and those practitioners who were supposed to assess them. The higher education ethos of the DipHE P2000 course was not relevant to the working reality of the ward. And because the orientation and quality of the ENB course 998 *Teaching and Assessing in Clinical Areas* varied in different centres, it was not unanimously considered helpful. That there were difficulties in assessing nursing students was supported by another study into assessment of diploma, degree and postgraduate levels in nursing and midwifery education (Gerrish, McManus and Ashworth, 1997). This work found a lack of clarity in the 'levels' students were expected to reach, both in their theory and in their practice, and noted inconsistencies in the educational frameworks used for such assessment.

Phillips, Schostak, Bedford and Leamon (1996), in another study, were more optimistic, but nevertheless, also found inconsistencies in the quality of support, teaching, facilitation and assessment. Some students expressed concerns:

> Actually a lot of the time mentors didn't really seem to understand some of the competencies but signed them anyway because they had to and because the university said they had to . . . "I don't know what the hell this means but I'll sign it anyway because you've been a good worker," nod, nod, wink wink, you know. So I'm sure I'm not the only one that's happened to.
>
> (Phillips et al., 1996: 111)

Teaching methods were primarily experiential, including self-direction and reflection, which was not only confusing and unstructured (Phillips et al., 1996: 119–21), but did not provide the knowledge and skills and 'nitty gritty' facts needed for confident practice:

> . . . there was a lot of stuff that I didn't feel that I knew . . . It was just silly things like how a certain pump works or how a certain insulin pen or something works . . . you can be fumbling with it for half an hour if you don't ask somebody.
>
> (Phillips et al., 1996: 170)

Another respondent wanted practical skills such as being able to give injections and perform catheterizations rather than 'psychological and social sorts of skills'. The researchers, however, argued that students should take responsibility for and create their own learning process and 'construct the essential sense of confidence' through individual interpret-ation; there were, after all, no objective 'facts' or 'skills' (Phillips et al., 1996: 171–72).

Uncertainty and fragmentation

The School Curriculum and Assessment Authority report (University of Exeter, 1996; SCAA, 1997) drew on the work of Gill Hek (1994) who found that only 9 per cent of institutions training nurses for Project 2000 required Mathematics GCSE grade C, and 54 per cent of colleges surveyed neither required nor preferred Mathematics as an entry criterion, nor looked for subjects reflecting numeracy (Hek, 1994). As the report commented: 'There is no homogeneity about mathematics entry for nursing' (University of Exeter, 1996: 7). Hek's results demonstrated that many colleges training nurses were concerned that the calculating skills of qualified nurses were very poor. None of the colleges she surveyed required A Levels, but all required GCSE qualifications or equivalent.

Whatever the difficulties of evaluating the new system (Wake, 1998: 242), there was consensus on one issue. Studies revealed uncertainty and fragmentation about what made for competency and how it was assessed. This finding was confirmed by two major studies published in 1997 (Luker, Carlisle, Riley, Stilwell, Davies and Wilson, 1997; May, Veitch, McIntosh and Alexander, 1997). The study on Project 2000 from Scotland found disparities between nurses' theoretical and practical knowledge. Furthermore, there may be some indication that nursing students were not happy with their training, for whatever reason, because there was an unacceptably high drop-out rate (May et al., 1997). Another study from Scotland in 1999 added to these concerns by finding inconsistency in student practical placement support, including some failures to adequately assess students' competence (Watson and Harris, 1999).

The study on nursing education for the Department of Health

The important study, produced by the Universities of Warwick and Liverpool for the Department of Health, concentrated on 'fitness for purpose' and the economic investment aspects of Project 2000 (Luker et al., 1997). The economic analysis broadly concluded that Project 2000 education and training was more costly than its predecessor, although it was too early to be definitive.

The part of the study concerned to discover whether nurses were fit for purpose used the method of individual and focus group interviews of managers at all levels, the latter to include nurses of 'F' grade upwards. The second strand of this part of the study was a national survey by questionnaire of newly qualified nurses. Evidence gathered from managers' opinions clearly pointed to problems. In their experience, managers found that, at registration, newly qualified nurses were not ready to practise and needed to consolidate training, even though according to the UKCC codes of conduct they were from that moment expected to be totally accountable and responsible for their practice. Clinical pressures and inadequate levels of experience among staff made this requirement of accountability problematic.

Although the researchers thought it was unfair to compare Project 2000 nurses with traditionally trained nurses (Luker et al., 1997: 46), they found serious problems voiced by managers. Managers had found themselves needing to shape the curriculum and not leave it to the college, if the nurses that were produced were to be fit for their purpose (Luker et al., 1997: 49). This apparently was not the case with nurses trained in the more traditional mode. Managers expected qualified nurses to have a knowledge base, definite clinical skills and certain personal qualities. They found Project 2000 nurses to be confident in challenging and questioning. That managers should see this 'in a positive light' was described by the researchers as 'heartening'; this undoubtedly fulfilled a basic tenet of the declared intention of the change in nurse education.

Managers who were *away* from clinical practice found nurses' confidence to be 'positive'. On the other hand, those managers with direct responsibility for patient care: 'were less likely to raise this as a positive quality without being prompted and a minority of managers felt that some of the diplomates had a potential for arrogance . . .'. There was disagreement about the quality of the new nurses' interpersonal skills. Nurses could not prioritize (Luker et al., 1997: 54–55). Nurses had difficulty translating what they had learned in theory to the clinical issues they faced in practice. The researchers wondered if this issue of competence in practice was actually a lack of confidence. Managers seemed to think so too, for they believed they had some responsibility for helping new nurses acquire practical skills (Luker et al., 1997: 59–61): 'They're lacking the skills and they know it' (Luker et al., 1997: 62).

Managers criticized the lack of practical core clinical skills, such as drug administration and injection technique and, in the case of mental health, the management of aggression. The managers 'were at pains to point out' other abilities such as research knowledge and care planning. Nevertheless, many nurses found difficulty with the idea of teamwork. The researchers interpreted the data in terms of managers having the wrong expectations: 'The changing structure of occupational roles in nursing is one which cannot be ignored in any study of "fitness for purpose"' (Luker et al., 1997: 63–66). And managers had failed to realize this.

This issue of changing roles was discussed. Managers considered whether they should rethink their expectations. Several managers thought the health care assistant could take over what was previously nursing work, and in particular, according to the researchers' description, 'dirty' tasks. Perhaps registered nurses would not need basic skills in future. But there was also an expression of 'an unhealthy scramble for tickets', an emphasis on academic attainment which devalued traditional nursing work and led to a feeling of threat amongst classically trained nurses (Luker et al., 1997: 66–71).

Managers knew little about the theoretical content of nurse education, regarded it as having insufficient practical placement involvement, and found the student's knowledge was often neither timely nor relevant. Moreover, managers felt that they needed to ensure new nurses were safe to practise, a point which nurses themselves echoed. They wanted more assessment of practice (Luker et al., 1997: 78–81).

Supernumerary students were now 'cosseted', unprepared for long hours and shift work. Their student experience was relaxed. They had freedom and learnt no discipline. Hence they could not handle responsibility. Particular concern was expressed about the clinical assessment of nursing skills (Luker et al., 1997: 93–97). Managers regretted that there were no formal assessments in Project 2000 as there had been in traditional nurse training. A number of managers were concerned about the diplomates' apparent lack of skill or knowledge in relation to drugs and drug administration. There was regret that the old certainties had gone:

> With the old assessments where you did a dressing or suturing or total patient care, but at least the tutor was there to go through it with them and give the guidance. Now I'm not saying that's by any means perfect, but at least there was someone identifiable who came and worked with the students. Now I think that something on that line would be beneficial.
>
> (Luker et al., 1997: 93)

Managers felt that practice staff were not supported by education staff in assessing students. Often clinicians' judgements were overturned or called into question. Many students had been able to successfully challenge clinicians' assessments, and trained staff felt that there was no way of 'failing a student'. Managers felt 'let down' by education staff (Luker et al. 1997: 95):

> I'm also certain that in order to achieve their (the college) objectives, some people are urged through that perhaps shouldn't be.
>
> (Luker et al., 1997: 96)

Luker et al. (1997: 125–36) distinguished between 'fitness for practice', deemed competency as laid down by statutory bodies, and 'fitness for purpose' according to the needs of the employer. They believed that the UKCC emphasis on theory might undermine the clinical skills needed by the employer. And the message to managers from Project 2000 was that such skills were not considered of value by educational establishments. A deep tension, between hospital needs and educational aims, is revealed.

However, they argued that employers were happy with the 'potential' if not the finished product, and they repeated their opinion that managers had 'a sense of optimism'. Yet the researchers admitted there were questions about the quality of care. They attempted to deal with these questions by referring to an article by While (1994), who suggested that what was required of a registered nurse should be linked to the concept of 'fitness for purpose' and actual performance in the practice setting rather than a more abstract concept of 'competence'. But, as the researchers point out, this is nebulous and still begs the question of defining what constitutes 'fitness for purpose', which is ultimately linked to the purpose of the role.

Managers were concerned about the 'practical skills illiteracy', but the researchers argued that managers seemed to expect newly qualified nurses to fit into 'old style roles and value systems', whereas roles were changing: 'change may need to take place with regard to the expectations of this new breed of staff nurse' (Luker et al., 1997: 135). The researchers questioned whether the new breed of trained nurses would actually be more like doctors, with health care assistants taking over traditional nursing tasks. The profession, they argued, needed to decide on the lines that would be drawn in distinguishing roles from health care assistant to doctor.

Accompanying the report was a letter by England's Chief Nursing Officer, Yvonne Moores, and Mike Deegan, the NHS Executive's Deputy Director (Moores and Deegan, 1997), which was sent to Trusts and Educational bodies, with copies to education groups and the UKCC and ENB. It announced the UKCC review of pre-registration education and training, which would also consider the report by Luker et al. The letter noted encouraging findings, and quoted phrases such as 'sense of optimism' and 'potential' used in the research by the researchers. The letter also noted the problems, realized the need to improve nurse training for the future, and noted the greater costs of Project 2000.

Moores and Deegan, therefore, made four suggestions for improvement: collaboration between the NHS and universities in clinical and academic settings; the improvement of skill acquisition by longer clinical placements and the use of a 'skills laboratory', and the improvement of teaching, supervision and assessment; the ensuring of preceptorship for newly qualified staff; and the creation of joint posts for teachers so that they could maintain links with clinical practice. Despite evidence to the contrary of serious problems in the preparation of nurses, Moores and Deegan concluded that Project 2000 had been successful.

Recognizing the problems of Project 2000

The interpretation of evidence in the study showed that the researchers were not neutral, disinterested or detached observers. The research was intended to highlight the strengths of Project 2000, as the researchers saw them, and to underplay the weaknesses. Value judgements were expressed throughout the report. Comments with which they were in favour were 'heartening', a value judgement used several times, and positive comments from managers about the effectiveness of Project 2000 came as a result of 'prompts'. This was to underplay the seriousness of the report's findings, for, as was noted by other researchers elsewhere, clinical experience undertaken without adequate training could lead to a potentially dangerous situation: '[clinical] experience without training increases confidence not competence' (McManus, Richards, Winder and Sproston, 1998: 348–49).

A feeling of confusion emanated from nurse education. The *Times Higher Education Supplement* quoted a trainee nurse specializing in mental health: 'I'm nearly finished now, but I feel completely unskilled . . . When I go on to acute admissions wards, I'm scared to death. I feel like a liability.' This underlined the finding from East Yorkshire Hospital NHS Trust that newly qualified staff lacked a grounding in essential clinical knowledge, and was typical of the general situation (Hinde, 1998: 6–7). This finding was further echoed in a study by Charnley (1999), who believed that there was a gap between the high expectations of newly qualified nurses and what they actually could offer. Charnley concluded that education should be more relevant to practice.

Further confirmation that standards for nurse preparation were now vague and haphazard was provided in a study by Neary (1999). Nursing students were continuously assessed during their common foundation programme to establish their clinical competence but many practitioners were ill-prepared to play the part of assessor, and students also realized this inadequacy. No formal system prepared assessors, and assessors worried about the level of their own competence. Preparation was '*ad hoc* and a waste of time' (Neary, 1999: 44). Both assessors and students expressed anger and frustration. Colleges had 'passed the buck' (Neary, 1999: 46) to practitioners for assessing the practical competence of nursing students, but practitioners did not feel competent to do this. They themselves wanted to be assessed. The study demonstrated the fragmentation and lack of communication there now was between the education establishments and clinical practice.

Project 2000 pre-registration courses did not keep students motivated. According to one study (Ghazi and Henshaw, 1998: 43–48), they were low attenders and poorly motivated in class. The reasons given were large group sizes, teacher shortages, a wide-entry gate, the course content and student-centred approaches. Some students had preconceived ideas based on the old curriculum of nurse education (by which the researchers appear to mean the national General Nursing Council syllabus), and they had difficulty with 'the broader approach of the new programme'. Students also had had little opportunity 'to control their own learning' and struggled with this approach.

The competence of the registered nurse

Competent to practise?

The competence of registered nurses was a matter of deep concern, according to many studies. A study by Bree-Williams and Waterman (1996) found that registered nurses were unsure about aseptic techniques for wound dressings. Cutting (1998) showed that registered nurses did not recognize infection in granulating wounds. Gould and Chamberlain (1997) discovered nurses' knowledge of routine infection control procedures to be patchy. Similarly, a study by Ridge, Jenkins, Noyce and Barber (1995) observed drug administration errors by nurses that were, in the authors' view, too high.

Todd, Freeman, Camilleri-Ferrante, Palmer et al. (1995) examined differences in mortality after hip fracture in an audit in East Anglia, and identified what they considered to be a high number of patients having pressure sores (22 per cent) and believed this to be 'noteworthy'. Although the study did not analyse the reason for this figure, pressure sore prevention was traditionally one of the most crucial nursing functions, and remained a prime test of nursing effectiveness (Cullum, Dickson and Eastwood, 1996).

Wilkinson (1996), in a survey of a thousand nurses, found widespread dissatisfaction with the level of education provided regarding the administration of intravenous therapy, and she quoted the Medical Devices Agency reports (1995a, 1995b) that there was a need among some sections of nursing for comprehensive training and education. Furthermore, one of the most common clinical procedures, blood pressure measurement, was also found to be problematic among nurses. A study by Gillespie and Curzio (1998) found that many nurses did not understand or perform the technique correctly, and recommended improvement in the learning and assessment of skills. A survey by a dental surgeon, a response to patients in a hospital and nursing homes who had received inadequate mouth care from nurses, found pre-registration nursing courses to be seriously lacking in oral hygiene teaching (Longhurst, 1998a and 1998b), a finding which supported an earlier study (Boyle, 1992; O'Dowd, 1998). Moreover, nurses were not taught first aid in pre-registration and post-registration courses (Godfrey, 1999); and medication education was haphazard (Latter, et al., 2000).

A confused curriculum

That nurses were now deficient in practical skills was related to the curriculum. Although nursing roles were extending, biomedical science was not being adequately taught in the pre-registration curriculum, and its quality was variable (Jordan and Potter, 1999). This in turn reflected a confusion about the nursing role and its preparation.

Hence, Smith, Masterson and Lloyd Smith (1999) found there to be a lack of clarity in British nurse education and practice about what constituted the nursing role, between 'health promotion versus disease and care'. Teachers, in their study, were glad to move away from disease-orientated philosophies of nursing, or 'forced to do so by the Project 2000 curriculum'. There was some quite severe dissonance. Students and ward-based practitioners expressed dissonance with the health promotion model; ward-based practitioners were strongly attached to disease-orientated models and with regard to health-promotion philosophies were 'beleaguered in tone' (Smith et al., 1999: 233). This was particularly problematic when students using a health promotion model of competence moved into clinical placements: 'Some lecturers claimed that clinicians' attitudes had compromised the educational goals of the College in meeting service needs (Smith et al., 1999: 236).'

According to the authors: 'Many Project 2000 students said they were dissatisfied with a health based curriculum because they had become nurses primarily to nurse sick people and not to promote health' (Smith et al., 1999: 236). The writers of this paper considered the dichotomy in nurse education and practice between health-orientated and disease-orientated philosophies of care to be of a factional nature – a clash of values. The clash of values also relates to the ambiguity about purpose, as studies by Luker et al. (1997), Robinson and Leamon (1999), and Smith et al. (1999) confirmed.

Similar problems were reflected in undergraduate degree nursing courses. With regard to content, particularly the biological sciences, Wharrad, Allcock and Chapple (1994) found great variation in the teaching of biological sciences on undergraduate nursing courses, particularly with regard to their relevance to nursing practice. Robinson and Leamon (1999), in a documentary analysis of nursing degree curricula, found it hard to differentiate graduate level practice from basic level practice as enshrined in rule 18A competencies. There was an extremely wide variation in curricula from different institutions, which made comparison of educational courses extremely difficult. Assessment of nursing practice was also arbitrary and inconsistent. Moreover, the general reliance on taxonomies of learning was highly questionable. The assessment of practical nursing skills was very variable. This finding was reinforced (Phillips et al., 2000; Bartlett et al., 2000).

Developing competence after registration?

Clinical supervision and PREPP

Perhaps clinical supervision by mentors and preceptors was envisaged as the way of ensuring that nurses once qualified would be competent. As pre-registration nursing documents made clear, nurse education was a process that did not end with qualification, and the UKCC's *Report of the Post-Registration Education and Practice Project* (PREPP) stated that newly registered practitioners needed to consolidate their competencies. Preceptorship was advocated as a means of support (UKCC, 1990: 18–19, para. 4). But here, too, the prevailing educational philosophy affected the meaning of 'supervision'.

As the report emphasized, 'individual practitioners when they register will have achieved specific competencies or learning outcomes and are accountable for their practice from the point of registration, regardless of any proposed support system' (UKCC, 1990: 18, para. 4.6). This point was further emphasized by the UKCC in discussing the period of support and preceptorship. The registered nurse was expected at the time of registration to be professionally competent and accountable at the minimum level of safety (Annexe 1 to Registrar's Letter 1/1993: 1; Registrar's Letter 3/1995: 2; Annexe 1 to Registrar's Letter 3/1995: 1). The preceptor was someone who helped the 'novice' nurse apply knowledge, integrate into the workplace and set learning objectives – offering support rather than assessment.

The concept of clinical supervision had grown out of the need to accommodate the philosophical changes in nursing from the biomedical to the interpersonal, and derived from a form of support known in psychology, social work and counselling. Supervision was not to be authoritarian but a form of peer-support and feedback, an enabling process encouraging 'personal and professional growth' (Butterworth, 1992: 9). Clinical supervision may also have been introduced as a scheme to 'stem the flow of people leaving the profession soon after registering' according to the PREPP executive summary: 'Clinical supervision is not a managerial control system. It is not a system of individual performance review and it should not be hierarchical in nature' (UKCC, 1997a: 8).

PREPP was not intended to introduce 'any form of restrictive practice' but it was seen as providing a 'blueprint' or 'encompassing framework for standards', the UKCC's 'central concern'. As the chairman wrote: 'The Council believes that, at the very least, minimum standards should be secured across the range of practice' (UKCC, 1990, Foreword). There seems to be a contradiction between this statement, that PREPP is a 'blueprint', and the statement of the chairman of the ENB that there was to be no 'blueprint' for nursing education (ENB, 1993b: 4).

But in reality PREPP was not intended to be prescriptive. The term 'blueprint' is used in the very vaguest of meanings. For while the UKCC emphasized that 'specific learning and updating is vital' following on from registration (UKCC, 1990: 10, para. 1.4) and that 'Competence can only be maintained by continuing education and professional development' (UKCC, 1990: 21, para. 5.1), the content of such education or the minimum standards of competence required of nursing practice were not prescribed.

Indeed, the proposed Personal Professional Profile, in which the practitioner recorded formal continuing education undertaken, involved 'a self-assessment of educational and developmental needs and a plan to meet these needs' (UKCC, 1990: 22, para. 5.9). The 'blueprint' was to be that there should be no 'blueprint'. PREPP proposals were finalized in 1994 (UKCC, 1994a) and accepted by the government, and known as PREP (UKCC, 1994b; UKCC, 1995). Standards for maintaining effective registration involved the requirement that a minimum of five days study should be undertaken every three years. The kind and content of the study was not prescribed, but included broad categories: reducing risk; care enhancement; patient, client and colleague support; practice development; and education development.

Practitioners were informed that the categories aimed to provide flexibility, personal and professional growth (UKCC, 1994b), and to ensure flexible, skilled professionals (UKCC, 1994a). The actual study days themselves were left up to the practitioner's own choice. There were to be no PREP-approved study days or formal requirements. This was emphasized by the UKCC: 'It is up to you how you wish to meet the study requirements' (UKCC, 1995: 3). PREP relied on self-appraisal, and according to the UKCC (1996b: 9) the council itself was still learning: 'There are no right or wrong answers to PREP.'

By 1998, concerned perhaps by the recruitment and retention crisis that had developed, the UKCC was to stress the ease by which PREP requirements could be met. Although nurses themselves were confused about how to meet PREP requirements, the UKCC, according to its policy development director, was to maintain its 'broad brush stroke' approach. PREP could be achieved in a variety of ways and there was to be no prescription: 'All we say is you should record your work in the way you feel most comfortable' (*Nursing Standard*, 1998l: 6). PREP requirements could be fulfilled by watching documentaries on television (*Nursing Times*, 1998h: 8). By the following year a report by management consultants KPMG for the UKCC found not only that nurses were not interested in and detached from PREP, but that the minimum requirements set by the UKCC were too low and irrelevant to practice. There was also a lack of clarity about how PREP requirements would be met (*Nursing Standard*, 1999a; M. Williams, 1999).

Growing concerns over the issue of nursing competence

Replacing prescription with flexibility

The new philosophy of nursing, ushered in by the 1979 legislation, rested on the belief that the previous nursing system was task-orientated and ritualized. As Chapter 1 has shown, under the old system nurses were taught to adhere to routines – the correct procedure for giving an injection, dressing a wound and laying up the dressing trolley, making a bed, treating pressure areas and preventing pressure sores, performing a bedbath, laying out the body after death. All this was detailed in nursing text-books, taught by tutors and ward sisters, documented in syllabuses and records of practical instruction and tested in practice and at final examination by GNC examiners. This traditional apprenticeship preparation was criticized as unthinking habits by which nurses were taught inflexibility and unquestioning obedience, for example, by Walsh and Ford (1989). The new system removed all such tasks and procedures. Nurses were now to be set free, encouraged to be creative, independent and flexible, but individually responsible for ensuring that whatever they did was based on 'evidence'.

The issue of competence seems to have become generally recognized as needing attention by 1997. Moves were already apparent from those who managed clinical practice. The Wellhouse NHS Trust, for example, 'were questioning how nurses would acquire competence to undertake new activities and how levels of achievement would be managed' (Fearon, 1998: 43). Various competencies that nurses needed were to be identified by the novice nurses themselves through self-assessment, and formal supervision and formative assessment provided. The nurse would then be graded in the particular skill (for example, intravenous therapy) in a detailed chart, rather in the manner of the old *Record of Practical Instruction and Experience*. Performance at different levels was assessed by marking the chart, which was signed by the assessor. This particular model of competency, however, was more detailed than that used in the previous system, as each activity was subdivided into separate steps. Competence for safe administration of intravenous medicines, as designed by the Wellhouse NHS Trust, had 17 categories or levels of performance in the one activity.

There was perceived to be a need for a rigorous method for defining, achieving and testing competence in particular skills. However, the issue still rested in the nurse's own self-awareness. Moreover, the system did not seem to have addressed skills deficits at the more basic level. It was hoped that this model of competence would increase 'personal awareness to recognize competence and limitations of practice' (Fearon, 1998: 45). It still relied on self-assessment, and for the nurse to be self-critical enough to recognize her limitations.

People initially identified as the supervisors were not nurses themselves but anaesthetists and phlebotomists. The NHS Trust recognized that no nurses were particularly expert in this field. The abandoned model of nurse training was brought to life by the Trust in more than the charting of skills and procedures. It was brought to life by employing the skills of doctors and other specialists in the teaching of nursing. This system was not part of educational or regulatory policy by the nursing bodies which were charged with the oversight of professional practice. Instead it was inaugurated by a Trust, on its own individual initiative, to address an unmet need: the need to prepare and assess nurses for clinical competence. Nevertheless, although this particular Trust put in a structure to help her, it was still left to the judgement of the individual nurse to decide, in the first place, what she needed to be able to do to be a competent nurse.

The UKCC recognition of incompetence

In 1996 the UKCC published *Issues Arising from Professional Conduct Complaints*. Complaints committees were confronted with professional misconduct in such areas as sexual harassment, theft, drug abuse, inappropriate delegation of responsibility, drug errors, improper restraint of patients and sexual relationships with patients. There were a significant number of cases referred to the UKCC where allegations related to the actual competence of the practitioner rather than professional misconduct. The UKCC admitted that there was no single act or omission serious enough to lead to removal from the register: 'The practitioner is really just not up to the required standard and may demonstrate a poor attitude, lack of insight and may make a number of errors over a period of time' (UKCC, 1996c: 7). But, 'the required standard' was a nebulous concept because, as the evidence has shown, there was no benchmark for determining this standard.

In March 1997 the nursing press reported on a UKCC seminar on incompetence. Forty-seven cases of incompetence had been thrown out because of gaps in legislation, and the professional conduct director of the UKCC, Mandie Lavin, suggested this was the tip of an iceberg: 'We have an undiagnosed potential epidemic . . . People know that we don't have the procedures to deal with this so maybe they don't report them to us' (*Nursing Times*, 1997b: 7; *Nursing Standard*, 1997b: 9).

In June of that year, *Nursing Times* reported on the UKCC council meeting. The UKCC was now considering a fundamental review of procedures to protect the public from incompetent nurses, midwives and health visitors. It wanted to issue managers with guidance on detecting incompetence and remind staff that they were accountable for their own competency levels and for reporting poor performances by colleagues. The UKCC did not have the power to remove incompetent practitioners and was seeking legal advice on how to tackle the issue. It needed, though, according to the report, to first agree a definition of incompetence, to research the link between poorly performing students and later incompetence, and establish how PREP could maintain competency levels. The council's professional officer, Hilary Jeffries, was reported as saying that new powers should be 'evidence-based' and command the support of the professions, and most importantly, promote higher standards of care (*Nursing Times*, 1997d: 6). The UKCC chief executive, Sue Norman, warned against a potential crisis in practice education. She said that nurses who had to do on-the-job training were not being given adequate support: 'I have serious concerns about the quality of practice education . . . We have to secure quality education and we have to reassure purchasers, the profession and the public that things are under control. We have a near crisis on our hands' (*Nursing Times*, 1997d: 6).

The government review of professional self-regulation of nursing

Reviewing self-regulation

It appears that the government was aware of concerns with nursing competence, because in March 1997 it commissioned an independent and fundamental review of the current operations of the five statutory bodies created by the Nurses, Midwives and Health Visitors Act 1979. The professional bodies submitted evidence to this review, conducted by JM Consulting, and sought to explain and justify shortcomings that were becoming apparent. JM Consulting issued a consultation document in January 1998 that considered the evidence (JM Consulting, 1998a), and issued its final report in August 1998 (JM Consulting, 1998b).

The UKCC evidence suggested that the move from the apprenticeship model of training to diploma-level education involved a diversion for the UKCC and National Boards. Their focus had been 'standards in education, particularly for nursing and health visiting, at the expense of standards in practice' (UKCC, 1997b: 4, paras.2.3, 2.4). Although the UKCC sought to justify its work, and used PREP as an illustration, it admitted that the standard, kind and content of pre-registration courses had been open to variable interpretation and implementation, and it suggested that this was because there were too many bodies involved in the educational process (UKCC, 1997b: 10, para. 5.2.4).

The ENB was also defensive (ENB News, 1997: 1; 1998a: 1; 1998c: 1,12), arguing that a 'key issue for the future will be the importance of ensuring that nurses, midwives and health visitors possess the knowledge and skills to practice (*sic*) competently on qualification and registration' (ENB News, 1999: 1). The RCN, however, appeared to argue for more flexibility, so that nurses could take on more roles and activities (*Nursing Standard*, 1998a: 6).

The review noted the changing nature of the nursing role, the lack of clarity of purpose in the statutory bodies and their members, and weaknesses in areas crucial to their prime purpose of public protection. These included lack of openness and transparency; and simple, consistent, equitable and comprehensible rules (JM Consulting, 1998a: 7, paras.

2.3–2.5). Although self-regulation was commended, the review also thought that the employer had an important role in supervision, mentoring, development and ensuring that practitioners remain fit to practise (JM Consulting, 1998a: 8–9, paras. 3.1–3.9). JM Consulting argued that a common regulatory scheme for all health professions would be desirable in the prime interests of patients (JM Consulting, 1998a: 10, paras. 3.10–3.13). The review suggested that the Act and statutory bodies should primarily be concerned with education of nurses and midwives 'to the point of registration; i.e. to ensure fitness to practise'.

According to the review, a newly qualified nurse would not be able to practise safely in every possible nursing situation but would be guided by supervision and the Scope of Professional Practice: 'to ensure safe practice by recognizing the limits of his or her competence and practising outside these' (JM Consulting, 1998a: 11, para. 3.15). Post-registration experience and accreditation went beyond statutory regulation (JM Consulting, 1998a: 11, para. 3.16). The Act ensured fitness to practise by conferring state registration on nurses and midwives deemed 'fit to practise'. Fitness to practise comprised appropriate educational qualifications, assessed clinical competence, health (the absence of physical or mental conditions that could harm patients), and professional conduct – suitable ethical standards and behaviour. This last, the review admitted, could not be guaranteed by any system of regulation (JM Consulting, 1998a: 14, para. 5.1).

According to JM Consulting there were 'notable weaknesses' in this regulatory system at present. These included the reluctance of many employers to check registration status; the relative lack of attention given to professional attitudes and standards in education programmes; the still imperfect integration of theory and practice education; and the feeling by many observers that practice education was given a lower priority than intended. There was also an inflexibility of powers available to the UKCC, and supervision was 'of variable quality and effectiveness' (JM Consulting, 1998a: 15, para. 5.4).

The review recommended that professional self-regulation should continue to depend on independent practitioners who acted in accordance with high-level definition of the scope of practice rather than on following detailed rules. Supervision should be supportive and developmental and a function of the employer (JM Consulting, 1998a: 15–16, paras. 5.6–5.8). The register should be simplified, higher qualifications should be recorded rather than registered, and registration status above the basic level should be based on clinical competence, which would include, but not be determined solely by, education qualifications (JM Consulting, 1998a: 17–18, paras.6.1–6.11).

JM Consulting suggested that the profession would need to debate the issue of defining and recording levels or qualifications based on the needs of public protection (JM Consulting, 1998a: 18–19, paras. 6.9–6.10). Education standards could be defined in terms of inputs (entry qualifications), process (curriculum, assessment methods) and outcomes (competencies required). The UKCC had a mix of the first and third and the National Boards contributed elements of the second. The review accepted that 'Many people agree that in general, regulatory bodies should be working towards outcome standards' (JM Consulting, 1998a: 19–20, paras. 7.7–7.9).

As regards the integration of theory and practice, the review noted the concern that the move from the NHS to higher education had led to an imbalance between the theoretical (or 'academic') part of training and the clinical practice component: 'They are intended to be of equal weight, but some observers complain that newly-qualified nurses are insufficiently confident in clinical situations.' One factor was claimed to be the lack of competence in higher education institutions in clinical education, 'and practical (or philosophical) difficulties in giving clinical experience sufficient priority in an educational institution'. The review rejected the suggestion of a pre-registration clinical year, and argued that education should be 'holistic or integrated'. The student should learn 'principles and new ways of thinking' from practice education in the workplace as well as in the classroom (JM Consulting, 1998a: 21, paras. 7.10–7.11).

The review touched on this issue in its next paragraphs, which focused on the relationship between higher education institutions (HEIs) and the regulatory bodies. The review noted that relations had not always been good: while some institutions welcomed the Boards, others found them to be unnecessarily heavy-handed and intrusive, 'as they (HEIs) have well-developed quality assurance systems and are capable of delivering nurse education without external scrutiny' (JM Consulting, 1998a: 21, para. 7.12).

And yet the review noted cases where HEIs had not understood their role in public protection: 'For example, there have been (isolated?) cases of unsuitable candidates accepted on "academic" criteria, or of clinical competence being down-graded in final assessments for academic award.' These difficulties, according to the review, resulted from perceived differences in the requirements of fitness for practice and fitness for award (JM Consulting, 1998a: 21, para. 7.13).

Project 2000 involved a 'huge' transfer of funds and according to JM Consulting it was not surprising that there were tensions. These occurred because of combining different disciplines with different values: health care and higher education. What did surprise JM Consulting, however, was the lack of broader debate at a strategic level around the changes of culture and values needed by the HEIs and the professions 'to achieve this desirable synthesis'. The review hoped that the Dearing Report (National Committee of Inquiry into Higher Education, 1997) would give added impetus to the debate with its focus on work-related learning (JM Consulting, 1998a: 21–22, para. 7.14).

Other health professions seemed to have found it easier and had developed strong centres of education and research led by the profession but distinct from the regulatory bodies. The RCN wanted to develop this role, but the review questioned this because it was a trade union. In the absence of such a centre, the UKCC and National Boards had sought to fulfil some of these functions, such as developing accreditation frameworks and undertaking research, but the review suggested that this function would be better delegated to a non-statutory body such as a faculty or academy (JM Consulting, 1998a: 22, para. 7.15).

In the view of JM Consulting, higher education institutions should be trusted. They 'could be relied upon to get the academic learning and quality assurance arrangements right'. It was the clinical placements that were problematic, and here the review suggested a greater number of practising clinicians rather than educationalists on the statutory bodies.

The review also considered whether the higher education Quality Assurance Agency would be able to take over the role of the National Boards, but noted that additional work would be needed to develop a framework for the assessment of clinical competence. As regards post-registration education, the review suggested that this should be developed by the professions, or by academic and research organizations rather than by statutory bodies (JM Consulting, 1998a: 22–23, paras. 7.16–7.19).

According to JM Consulting, the regulatory body should move from being punitive and rule-bound to being more developmental and enabling. It questioned whether the UKCC had a strategy for conduct standards, whether it gave clear guidance, whether its powers and sanctions were adequately flexible, whether more lay people should be involved in disciplinary committees, and whether there should be more dialogue with employers and complainants and more openness in the decisions made (JM Consulting, 1998a: 24–26, paras. 8.1–8.13). With regard to the structure of the statutory bodies, the review suggested a new, unified system of professional self-regulation (JM Consulting, 1998a: 27–29, paras.9.1–9.10).

Finally the report considered the support worker, whose numbers had made them a large group, and who took on a significant proportion of what in the past would have been regarded as nursing tasks. The growth of the support worker had occurred because of the difficulty in recruiting trained nurses, the need for cost effectiveness, and access and flexibility: '. . . many caring and dedicated people wish to work in a health care role but for a number of reasons may be unable or unwilling to undertake the full preparation as a registered nurse, or to work the hours and responsibilities that this demands (these include some former nurses)' (JM Consulting, 1998a: 33, paras. 12.1–12.2).

The support worker was supposed to work under the supervision of the trained nurse, but it was argued to be unsafe to ask nurses to delegate functions to staff who might have no qualifications and no checks on their character or employment history. The review recommended some check on character, particularly a criminal record, and a basic qualification (NVQ or occupational standard). But it thought regulation would be difficult and should be left as the responsibility of the employer (JM Consulting, 1998a: 33–34, paras. 12.3–12.8).

The responses to JM Consulting's review

In response, the RCN advocated permissive approaches to regulation, and an enabling, empowering approach to regulation. It called for the permissiveness of current legislation to be the approach enshrined in future statute (RCN, 1998a: 5, paras. 3.1–3.4). The RCN agreed that the move into higher education had presented a problem of combining fitness for purpose (clinical competence, confidence and professional autonomy) with the fitness for award (diploma or degree). In its view a future higher education Quality Assurance Agency should take on course approval currently undertaken by National Boards, and local regulatory organizations could concentrate on clinical placements, supervision and competence accreditation.

The RCN saw itself as having an important future role in shaping professional standards and coordinating 'an independent professional voice for nursing' (RCN, 1998a: 16, paras. 9.7–9.9). It also suggested that employers should be responsible for assessing incompetence at the workplace to ensure that the individual appeared to be competent at the basic level of registration (RCN, 1998a: 22, para. 11.4).

The ENB response affirmed the importance of standards and argued that it had set up a new quality assurance framework to replace the revalidation of programmes with monitoring and review. This would clarify respective responsibilities of the ENB and higher education institutions. It strongly disagreed with JM Consulting's view that 'much of the work in developing education standards and measures of clinical competence could desirably be taken forward outside the regulatory system'. The ENB argued that these aspects were at the heart of professional regulation and best addressed by the regulatory system charged with ensuring the achievement and maintenance of the standards (ENB, 1998a: 12).

If these review recommendations were accepted, the boards were to be limited to a role in clinical placements and accreditation of clinical competence, and the ENB argued that the review was simplistic in its approach to standards and levels of practice, and did not understand professional quality assurance (ENB, 1998a: 10–13, paras. 7.3–7.15; *Nursing Times*, 1998b: 6). The ENB dismissed the proposal of JM Consulting that a 'simple statement of education standards' was possible to ensure competence and so protect the public (ENB, 1998a: 13, para. 7.15).

The ENB rejected the idea of creating an academy and delegation of post-registration frameworks to it, believing this would fragment frameworks for continuing competence (ENB, 1998a: 14, para. 7.16). But it also called for more in-depth consideration of unregulated health care assistants, recognizing that 'An increasing number of unregulated healthcare personnel provide direct patient/client care, often with the most vulnerable sections of the society' (ENB, 1998a: 18, para. 12.1).

The ENB published the *Quality Assurance Manual* in 1998, which set out the framework for institutions going through the process of validation for professional regulation. It sought to address the requirement of 'Fitness for purpose, practice and award' (ENB, 1998c: 5), but like earlier ENB publications, this new document contained no detailed standards of competence expected from registered nurses.

The final report of JM Consulting was published in August 1998 (JM Consulting, 1998b). In the light of its review and the findings of its consultation document, it recommended that a new regulatory body should define standards for nurse education in terms of outcome and fitness to practise, should develop policies to ensure outcomes were achieved, and should ensure institutions were accredited to an appropriate standard (JM Consulting, 1998b: 15, paras. 74–76). The report found clinical supervision to be anomalous and variable, and recommended that the new Council should have discretionary powers to make rules for statutory supervision (JM Consulting, 1998b: 21, paras. 100–104). The report appears to have been a recognition and admission that nursing preparation needed rigorous improvement if nurses were to be competent.

The UKCC Commission on nurse education

The UKCC responded to the government review proactively, by setting up its own commission to look at practical training needs of nurses. The UKCC Commission was, moreover, designed to look into the future of nurse education (*Nursing Times*, 1998c: 6), just over a decade since Project 2000 had been accepted by government. The cost of this would be £500,000 and there were as yet no terms of reference. Terms of reference were published subsequently. These stated that the commission was to prepare a way forward for pre-registration nursing and midwifery education that enabled fitness for practice based on health care need, with particular regard to: 'the contemporary and anticipated needs of health care; an outcomes based competency approach to fitness for practice; sound assessment of practice and its integration with theory; the nature of and standards for the teaching of nursing and midwifery; and positioning in relation to possible inter-professional approaches where appropriate'. Importantly, the commission would use existing evidence, building on work already done, 'and will only commission additional work that cannot be found elsewhere or is insufficient for the Commission's needs (UKCC Education Commission, Terms of Reference, 1998b). The implications were clearly that assessment of practice, standards of teaching, and competency, were not forming a currently satisfactory basis for making nurses 'fit for practice'.

The UKCC chose as chairman for its commission, Sir Leonard Peach, NHS chief executive from 1986 to 1989, in post during the period of the government's acceptance of Project 2000 and its subsequent implementation. The UKCC Commission was to survey 80,000 students and staff for their opinions and perceptions. It was keen to understand the high student drop-out rate (*Nursing Standard*, 1998h). But how open-minded and impartial would the commission be in its analysis of the evidence? The UKCC head of communications (Skyte, 1998: 52–53) commended Project 2000 and denied that by setting up the commission inferences of criticism could be drawn. Similarly, he dismissed 'the common fallacy' that academic education reduced practical skills. But the very fact that the UKCC was now considering whether pre-registration education should be competency based, and what level of academic or vocational qualification was required, showed all was not well. Moreover, the UKCC was doing further research into student attrition from pre-registration courses and the level of preparedness of new entrants to the profession. The UKCC did not want to admit it, but it undoubtedly recognized severe concerns. Paradoxically, so did a nursing professor, a powerful advocate for academic nursing (Clark, 1998: 54), who thought that nurse education was now 'an inglorious mess – full of anomalies, perverse incentives and conflicting goals'.

The person selected to chair the commission, Sir Leonard Peach, was involved with Project 2000 from its earliest days, and therefore had a vested interest in its preservation and continuation. An interview with him in the *Nursing Standard* (Lipley, 1998: 14) raises the question of his objectivity. Peach stated that he was not convinced by what he called 'hearsay' evidence, that because newly qualified nurses lacked confidence this confirmed speculation by many in the health service that Project 2000, with its emphasis on academic education, had sent nurse training down

the wrong route. He argued that education and willingness to learn made
nurses so adaptable to change that they could even move on to other
professions outside nursing. Transferable skills meant nurses 'can go into
other similar professions or careers in management'. This itself is an
ironical conclusion given the then current recruitment crisis, which he
also did not accept.

The questionnaire sent to registered nurses by the commission was
revealing of a deep concern. Questions from this attitudinal survey,
conducted by BMRB International, asked how well the registrant 'thought'
pre-registration education prepared newly qualified nurses for their areas
of practice (UKCC Commission, 1998a). Following questions asked the
respondent to 'assess' nurses educated by Project 2000 with regard to
knowledge, questioning, communication, confidence, relating theory to
practice, motivation to learn, problem-solving, practical skills, teamwork
and management. What was the respondent's 'opinion' of the balance of
theory and practice on current pre-registration courses? Were students
provided with enough support from teaching staff to link theory with
practice? Were newly qualified staff supported by a named practitioner?
Attitudes to patients were not specifically included, so there was no
attempt to find out whether nurses were prepared for compassion and
'caring'. But the nature of the survey indicates that it was questionable
whether newly qualified staff were prepared in even the most basic ways
for practice.

That the ENB also recognized the current failings in nursing education
was made clear by its evidence to the UKCC Commission. The ENB
evidence to the commission (ENB News, 1999: 8) included recommendations that students should have earlier clinical experience; that national
core competencies should be identified; that theory and practice should
be integrated; and that preparation of mentors, supervisors and assessors
should be improved.

Problems in nursing education were now recognized. The UKCC
Commission published its report on nurse education in 1999 (*Nursing
Times*, 1999c). The open-mindedness of the commission to change was
an important question. The report was prefaced by the chairman, Sir
Leonard Peach, who described his own part in the introduction of Project
2000: 'In addition, in the 1980s, I had been privileged to play a part in the
approval of Project 2000 . . .' (UKCC, 1999a: 1). The assumption running
through the report was that radical change was unnecessary and even
unthinkable.

Although the report stated its basis in a large weight of evidence, the
evidence was not produced in the report in any form that could be
objectively analysed. Rather, statements referred to secondary sources,

research studies, and were interspersed with findings from the attitude survey and consultation gatherings that the UKCC had undertaken. So, for example, the report stated that many educational institutions offered 'flexible and innovative' programmes (UKCC, 1999a: 2, para. 13). But no evidence was given to support this statement, or indicate what was meant by it. Moreover, some statements would seem to be contradicted by available and published evidence not taken account of in the report.

Similarly, the report stated that respondents to its consultations were generally positive about the move of schools and colleges into higher education and appreciated the broader-based theoretical preparation covering social sciences and biological sciences. Managers interviewed appreciated the course content as now including social sciences (UKCC, 1999a: 40, para. 4.38). No comment was made about the concerns that biological sciences were marginalized, which by the time of the report was admitted by researchers in this area (Smith et al., 1999). Perhaps this was because many teachers working in higher education were present at the consultations. Indeed, the report did not make any systematic analysis of, or indeed reference to, the curriculum content as it was taught to nurses at all. It is difficult, therefore, to judge against evidence the objectivity or accuracy of the statements made by the report, and which formed the basis for its judgements and recommendations. The UKCC used evidence from its attitude survey that many new nurses felt confident after a period in a new post (UKCC, 1999a: 43, para. 4.57). But this would seem to be unreliable evidence of actual competence, as has been suggested by McManus et al.(1998).

The report admitted that the commission set out with an assumption that 'diversity is a strength, and we did not wish to undermine it by making detailed, prescriptive recommendations', although a common approach was recognized to be needed (UKCC, 1999a: 2, para. 13). The report did admit serious weaknesses with nurse education. Not only was there a fragmentation of theory and practice, and inadequate supervised practical experience for students, but core competencies were not defined. There was a vagueness and lack of clarity in assessment of competence (UKCC, 1999a: 37, paras. 4.20–4.21). There were, the report implied, no clear standards. One recommendation was to define these.

The report sought to ascribe such failures as a failure not of principle, but of implementation (UKCC, 1999a: 3, para. 19). It recommended the move towards outcome-based competencies, which would need to be defined, and which working groups were already considering. The commission took account of purported limitations of outcomes-based education as bureaucratic, restrictive and reductionist, and marginalizing academic skills and abilities such as analysis, synthesis, ingenuity and creativity. In line with its own non-prescriptive approach, it therefore advocated a 'liberal or broad interpretation of competency'. Outcomes could be defined, the commission believed, 'which do not control the curriculum in such a way that restricts understanding, freedom of thought or originality' (UKCC, 1999a: 35–36, paras. 4.12–4.13). Graduate expansion was recommended (UKCC, 1999a: 33, para. 3.68).

Despite its own work in seeking to define future need for health care (Warner, Longley, Gould and Picek, 1998), the commission admitted that there was no consensus on the nursing role; nor did it seek to define one (UKCC, 1999a: 44, paras. 4.62–4.63). The UKCC had at last recognized the problems in nurse education, in reaction to government criticism, but the report was superficial in both its evidence and analysis, with the consequence that it failed to grasp the nettle of defining precisely what the nursing role was and would be, and what standard of competence was required to fit that role.

As the press reported, the commission admitted there were shortcomings (*Nursing Times*, 1999e; *Nursing Standard*, 1999c). There was a gulf between theoretical and practical elements of training, according to the chief executive, Sue Norman: 'There has been a fracturing between the academic and practical components of training' (*Nursing Times*, 1999e: 5). It is interesting that the word 'training' rather than 'education' was used – a reversion to a term that had been discouraged by the modern academic approach to nurse preparation. But, most importantly, there was a recognition that standards of competence needed definition now, that nurses' practical skills needed developing and monitoring, and there was acceptance that nursing should not be an all-graduate profession. The UKCC hoped, however, that 'tweaking' the system rather than radical overhaul would satisfy criticisms. The *Guardian*'s social services correspondent, David Brindle (1999c: 9), wondered if the government would want a more thorough change. The government response will be considered in Chapter 6.

The consequences of Project 2000 on the influence of the ward sister

The new system of nurse preparation had brought fragmentation into the curriculum as individual institutions designed their own courses, so that the former national system by which nurses in all parts of the country followed the same syllabus and were trained to the same standard was lost. It also moved the curriculum away from biomedicine, the involvement of doctors in teaching, and the standardized learning of practical skills.

But not only the nature of the curriculum and mode of education changed with the introduction of Project 2000. Most significantly, studies and reports on the effectiveness of nurse education paid virtually no attention to the role of the ward sister in both the education of the nurse and the supervision of the standards of practice. This was because the ending of the apprenticeship system ended *ipso facto* the predominating influence of the ward sister's role. There were three significant factors in the change.

First, the separation of nurse education from service to patients, which was the central intention behind the new educational system, had deep consequences for practice, specifically on the ward sister's position. Under the former apprenticeship system, the ward sister had been responsible for teaching and supervising student nurses, inducting them into the ethos of care, and ensuring the quality of the care that patients received on her ward. Under the new system nurses were taught in colleges, and mentored on the wards by their peers.

Second, by transferring autonomy and accountability for patient care from the ward sister to the individual registered nurse, the ward sister was effectively demoted from her former responsibility for standards of nursing practice and patient care. Individual nurses were responsible for their own allocated patients and for their own individual actions.

Third, the culture of autonomy affected ward coherence. Flattened hierarchy had replaced the former clearly defined hierarchy and chain of responsibility, which had involved doctors, matrons and ward sisters. The mutual interdependence of the previous system, within which the ward sister was the fulcrum, was replaced by the independence of individual autonomous practitioners. As a consequence the community of relationships known as professional etiquette was fragmented, and the ward sister as ward leader was disempowered.

These three factors meant that the ward sister's sphere of influence was profoundly diminished with regard to the development of moral character, ward-based practical learning, the supervision of patient care, and her role as the pivot of ward relationships, known formerly as professional etiquette. Nurses were no longer inducted into this ethos. The four principles of the former apprenticeship tradition had become entirely irrelevant to the new system.

Conclusion

Professional leaders had sought a new structure for education befitting new forms of self-regulation. Trust was placed in the individual learner to take responsibility for his or her own learning. It was thought the nursing student would be self-motivated, self-developing, creative, flexible and self-critical; but this proved to be questionable. For how did the nurse know what she or he did not know? There was now no national syllabus or set of procedures: nurse preparation had become virtually a liberal arts education with very little orientation or induction into practical nursing and the discipline needed for service to patients. One illustration serves as an example: mouth care, prescribed in detail under the former system, was found to be extremely haphazard under the new system.

Education now defined service, rather than, as in the previous system, service defining education. The removal of nurse preparation from service requirements had implications for patient care. There was an impasse between the philosophy underpinning the new educational preparation for nursing, and the reality of what was needed from nurses by patients and clients. The central question would be whether nurses were fitted to address these needs. A significant factor was the diminishing of the ward sister's role as teacher, supervisor and leader. By 1999 it was clear that there were some fundamental problems with nurse education, as even the UKCC admitted, even though major change was rejected *a priori*. Nevertheless, the purpose of the nurse, the nursing role and function, would become the key issue, as following chapters will show.

CHAPTER 4

'Professionhood', vocation and new nursing roles 1990–1999

Introduction

Because education had now come to define service, so the needs of service in relation to nursing roles were redefined. The new policy for the nursing profession established in the wake of Project 2000 brought a profound shift in ethos and culture, and this chapter will chart the way this affected the professional nursing role. The traditional caring role became less prestigious as basic caring values lost esteem in the late twentieth century, and practical care became synonymous with low status work. Basic caring was parted from high technology caring. Nursing became dualistic. New expanded nursing roles achieved higher status and were seen as the way to advance the profession, and the task of personal bodily care was left to unqualified staff. But many nurses and other commentators still sought to retain the vocational tradition and its values, which made apparently 'low status' work of inestimable value and the core of nursing.

Changing values: caring now out of date?

The closing decade of the twentieth century marked a decline in regard for basic caring. Altruism in society generally was considered to be waning. Evidence for this was given by the *British Medical Journal*, which reported a qualitative study about the decline in altruism and the threat to blood supplies. Young people especially had a strong resistance to 'doing good' (Ferriman, 1998: 1405). As one respondent was quoted: 'I have other ways of feeling good, rather than helping other people. I like to go out with my friends, and I like to drink a lot of beer. I like to sit and watch TV. I'm not always helping other people.' The decline in altruism might also have had consequences for nursing recruitment. The 'postmodern' trend in society revealed itself in such surveys.

This purported decline in altruism was illustrated by a study of young people aged 10, 15 and 17 for the Department of Health, which examined their perceptions of nursing as a career. The study found that caring was regarded negatively, except if it was for young children or animals (Foskett and Hemsley-Brown, 1998). According to the researchers, adolescents are naturally self-obsessed and the notion of caring for others more than themselves was unattractive. 'Helping' was considered a more active idea. Caring was considered to be passive, unassertive, feminine, involving the 'rather outdated notion of "self-sacrifice"', as well as 'friendly', 'loving' and 'dedicated'. Nurses were thought to offer emotional support rather than clinical expertise (Foskett and Hemsley-Brown, 1998: 28–29, para. 3.5.1), and were considered to be 'subservient' to doctors (Foskett and Hemsley-Brown, 1998: 46, para. 4.5). Children were squeamish and did not like the idea of blood or death (Foskett and Hemsley-Brown, 1998: 31–35, para. 3.5.3).

Although 17-year-olds appreciated that nurses were 'well qualified' and 'well educated' (Foskett and Hemsley-Brown, 1998: 52, para. 4.7), they saw little advantage in studying nursing at university but would rather aim higher by becoming doctors: 'If both nursing and medicine (to become a doctor) require a degree they argue that they may as well study medicine' (Foskett and Hemsley-Brown, 1998: 50, para. 4.6). Interestingly, low pay does not seem to have been a major factor in the reason for not choosing nursing as a career – lack of interest was the main reason (Foskett and Hemsley-Brown, 1998: 24–26, para. 3.4). Nursing as a career was seen as a 'customary' job, in contrast to the nature and role of a doctor which was regarded as a 'high status' job (Foskett and Hemsley-Brown, 1998: 85, para. 5.4).

The researchers' conclusion was that promotional literature aimed at young people should address and go beyond these negative perceptions. Nursing should be described in 'gender neutral' terms, and the feminine bias removed. The 'over-emphasis' on caring should be readjusted to concentrate on helping by presenting specialist areas, particularly children's nursing and midwifery. Images should be of intellectual knowledge required, teamworking, and avoidance of comparison with doctors. Nurses should be seen in an 'assertive advisory role', working at practical tasks that avoided injections or open wounds, and in 'practitioner' roles. Positive outcomes of nursing should be emphasized rather than operations or death. Subtle ways of promoting 'male niches' in theatre nursing should be developed, for example, by a medical emphasis and reducing the caring element (Foskett and Hemsley-Brown, 1998: 90–92, para. 6.3). The researchers admitted that the government advertising campaign had followed this approach (Foskett and Hemsley-Brown, 1998: 89, para. 6.2), although they do not mention that despite this campaign recruitment had at that time reached crisis point.

Much of Foskett and Hemsley-Brown's data came from focus groups, and it is a matter for speculation to what extent answers from the young people were subjected to influence. Certainly it is strange that when questioned about nursing as a career choice ten-year-old boys giggled, although older boys and middle-class boys were, in the words of the researchers, more conscious of being careful to be 'politically correct' in their responses:

> Some boys tried to argue that nursing is only for women and although they were always challenged in the focus group by other boys, it was clear that this view was underlying their bemused reactions.
> (Foskett and Hemsley-Brown, 1998: 40–41, para. 4.2)

Whereas the researchers were keen to promote an image of nursing that they thought would appeal to young people, for example by reducing the 'caring' or 'squeamish' aspects, they did not suggest appealing to the gender bias of the young: instead they sought to challenge this assumption. It is noteworthy that several children did mention 'care' or 'caring' in relation to nursing. The authors admitted this (Foskett and Hemsley-Brown, 1998: 27–29, para. 3.5.1), but they were keen to make a distinction between 'helping' and 'caring'. Indeed, the view of caring associated with 'self-sacrifice', expressed in focus group sessions, was qualified by the authors as 'a rather outdated notion'.

Whether the children questioned or interviewed themselves assumed such a distinction in the language they used, and, moreover, whether their opinions were subject to verbal and non-verbal influences, is open to question. Nevertheless it is clear that the researchers brought their own perspectives to the interpretation of their study. They believed that in order to attract recruits, the passive 'caring' image of nursing should be downplayed in favour of a more active 'helping', and that the focus should be 'intellectual' rather than 'physical'. The intrinsic value of 'basic nursing care' was shown to be unpopular and distasteful.

These findings, that children had negative perceptions of a career in nursing, were echoed in a research study carried out by David Bullivant (1998: 10). Schoolchildren expressed physical and psychological barriers to nursing, including 'squeamishness'. They also thought nurses to be low in status although they were 'nice compassionate people'.

Confusion over the nursing role?

The health care assistant and personal nursing care

This argument over the status of nursing in relation to tasks of personal care predominated during the last decade of the twentieth century. In 1992, at an RCN conference, there were murmurings of discontent at the suggestion that in order to improve its image nursing ought to drop its low-status work. Nursing had rejected its angel image, was aiming to be a highly qualified profession, and had assumed more obligations, which included some responsibility for diagnosis. But arguments followed that nurses were pricing themselves out of the market (Dean, 1992). Their work was gradually being taken over by health care assistants.

The rise in the number of health care assistants became a feature of the 1990s, as might have been predicted by the removal of student nurses from the nursing workforce. This is clear from two reports published by Unison. *Condition Critical* (Unison, 1997), a survey of 1,338 nurses, midwives and health visitors prepared as evidence to the 1998 Nurses, Midwives and Health Visitors Pay Review Body, found that many were considering leaving the nursing and midwifery professions altogether. Forty-five per cent considered there was a fall in the quality of care, and over half of ward sisters and senior staff nurses thought this was the case. Eighty-eight per cent of all nursing staff (nine out of ten) agreed that nurses and midwives were taking on work previously performed by doctors. Over three quarters of all nursing grades thought that non-registered staff were now performing duties previously performed by registered staff.

The second study published by Unison, *The Invisible Workers*, was carried out by Carole Thornley, Lecturer in Industrial Relations, Department of Human Resource Management and Industrial Relations, University of Keele (Thornley, 1997a), who also published an article on it in *Nursing Times* (Thornley, 1997b). Thornley found that the policy towards the greater use of nursing support workers (health care assistants as they later became known) from the mid-1980s was seen in different ways by the government and the nursing profession.

Nursing 'professionalisers', said Thornley, did not see eye to eye with the government. The former wanted the role to be strictly limited and clearly distinguished from 'nursing' while the government perceived a much greater role for a new 'trained' grade with clear and direct responsibility for patient care. The government also thought this might lead to eventual entry into nurse training or 'equivalent' nursing grades (Thornley, 1997a: 4).

The government had been in favour of the support worker. As John Moore, then Secretary of State for Health, wrote to Audrey Emerton, Chairman of the UKCC, the government's agreement to the introduction of Project 2000 rested in the important contribution to be made to the provision of care by greater use of the support worker role. Indeed, Moore's successor as Secretary of State for Health, Kenneth Clarke, also wrote to Audrey Emerton affirming the use of support workers, but suggesting that in order to avoid confusion between qualified nurses and support workers, who could include ward clerks, ward orderlies, receptionists and so on, the title 'health care assistant' should be used in place of 'support worker', a term which was 'inelegant and less descriptive'. Clarke also expressed concern at the lack of clarity about the respective roles of qualified nurses and support workers (Clarke, 1989, 1399A, paras. 10–11).

According to Thornley (1997a) health care assistants' work content showed that they were undertaking many duties previously performed by nurses, but with varying degrees of supervision. Health care assistants talked to/reassured patients and relatives (97 per cent); made beds (86 per cent); helped bathe patients (83 per cent); liaised on the telephone with patients, relatives and departments (83 per cent); monitored/ recorded patient observations (82 per cent); helped feed patients (79 per cent); obtained specimens (78 per cent); helped with catheter care (61 per cent); participated in meetings about patient care (57 per cent); performed dressings and wound care (57 per cent); assisted in drawing up care plans (43 per cent); handled syringes/equipment (43 per cent); helped with drug administration (42 per cent); performed clinical stock control (37 per cent); performed invasive procedures (18 per cent); and took blood samples (11 per cent). Fifteen per cent did other tasks not listed.

Just over a tenth of health care assistants surveyed said 'all' or 'some' of their work was supervised, 35 per cent said 'some' of their work was supervised and the majority (53 per cent) said 'little' or 'none' of their work was supervised. The main strength of feeling was that not enough training, particularly off-job training, was provided although, as the report notes, 25 per cent thought that they had the 'right amount' of training provided. Only 30 per cent of health care assistants had acquired a National Vocational Qualification (NVQ).

Thornley built on this work in a further report for Unison published the following year (Thornley, 1998a and 1998b), when she looked at the work of nursing auxiliaries and assistants. She found that not only did they perform the greater part of front-line personal care for patients, for whom they had the time that trained nurses did not, but nearly two-thirds engaged in at least one of the following duties: liaising with doctors; cardiac massage; helping train students or newly-qualified nurses; setting up/monitoring diagnostic machines; supervising staff; providing care of patients in their own homes; setting up drip feeds; taking charge of shifts. A small number gave injections. In fact, the work content of health care assistants and nursing auxiliaries was almost identical in percentage terms. Similarly, nursing auxiliaries and assistants had little or no supervision. And just over one third had attained an NVQ. Yet, Thornley (1998a: 19) argued, it was a misunderstanding to refer to nursing auxiliaries as 'untrained' or with 'very limited training', because many were experientially trained through 'learning on the job'.

Further work by Thornley in 1999 continued to show unqualified ancillaries, health care assistants and auxiliaries running wards. In a national survey of 250,000 staff in UK hospitals, she found that hospital managers, in the face of budget deficits and major shortages of registered nurses, were turning to unqualified ancillaries to staff wards (Thornley, 1999).

The editor of the *British Journal of Nursing* commented on the first Unison report:

> It seems that nursing is totally confused. The hypocrisy of this system wherein the HCA [health care assistant] does the true nursing without the guidance of the UKCC or the protection of the RCN or the structure of further education is obvious.
>
> (Scott, 1997: 1092)

Concerns about unqualified care workers taking on more nursing roles was evident also in a report on children at home (NHSE, 1998c). One of the major conclusions of the report was that because nurses seemed to be taking on more of a supervisory role, care staff without formal nursing qualifications were carrying out complicated nursing procedures in the home: 'Questions were raised on the safety of such practice, the training provided and responsibility' (NHSE, 1998c: 34, para. 6). The report elucidated some confusion concerning 'What is a nursing duty?', and the growing trend to use health care assistants to carry out duties that formerly would have been done by registered nurses (NHSE, 1998c: 8, para. 1.52).

In Parliament, Labour MP Audrey Wise expressed concerns in a Commons health committee about unqualified care assistants taking over nursing work. She thought that tasks such as bathing enabled nurses to pick up problems when they were easier to treat (Wise, in House of Commons, 25 February 1998a: 12–14). Wise's opinion was supported by evidence. Carr-Hill, Dixon, Gibbs et al. in 1992 had performed a study which found that quality of care improved when qualified nurses performed it. 'Care' for the researchers included such matters as patient hygiene, patient nutrition and hydration, pressure sores/skin integrity, intravenous therapy, planning for patient discharge, pain control, education/rehabilitation and elimination (Carr-Hill et al., 1992: 31–32, para. 3.3.2).

It seems that pragmatic considerations continued to hold sway, however. In 1998, *Nursing Times* (1998e: 6) reported that Swindon and Marlborough NHS Trust, with the assent of the local Labour MP, Julia Drown, was replacing nurses with care assistants in order to cut the budget. This was occurring in a political climate which was set to impose on Trusts the duty to monitor and audit standards of patient care (*The New NHS*, 1997). Hence, it must be assumed that the Trust did not believe that care would suffer adversely by its actions. Care assistants were becoming nurses in all but name.

An all-graduate profession?

Meanwhile, professional leaders were seeking to make nursing education more academic, and arguing for an all-graduate profession (Clark, 1997; Council of Deans and Heads, 1998). The UKCC also accepted the case for graduate entry. The Council President, Mary Uprichard was reported as saying: 'In my view we have undersold and undervalued nursing by not having entry at graduate level' (*Nursing Times*, 1997a: 9). And the RCN published a discussion document, *Shaping the Future* (RCN, 1997c), which recommended that nursing should indeed become an all-graduate profession. A paper by Traynor and Rafferty (1998) reinforced the notion that such a desired change must rest on revised nursing values.

But not all nurses agreed. In the *British Journal of Nursing* a correspondent commented on the RCN discussion document. Although it might seem surprising to suggest a complete overhaul of nurse education so soon after the last radical change, she and her colleagues were not surprised. But this appeared to be for very different reasons to those underpinning the document itself. For while the document sought more integration with higher education by complete graduate status for the nursing profession, this correspondent, Janice Barrett, a registered nurse, deplored the weaknesses of the present college-based system.

From her own 'old-style' training she had become a competent nurse aware of her limitations and capabilities: 'I now work with many new diplomates and graduates and realize how difficult and inappropriate their training has been. While they are experts on some academic aspects of nursing, they lack the ability to put this theory into practice'. Practical experience, which was so crucial to competence, had been cut to a minimum (Barrett, 1997: 1136).

Similarly, the Head of Workforce Planning and Education (Nursing and PAMs) at the NHS Executive, Gill Newton, raised her concerns about this proposal to replace diploma courses by degree courses (Newton, 1998: 62). First, she envisaged recruitment to be a problem. At present the number of applications for each diploma place was lower than a few years ago (1.2 applications per place). Would potential candidates be put off if diversity of preparation was not maintained? Second, would a new tier of worker need to be recruited to do the work that graduate nurses were unwilling or unavailable to do? Third, Newton predicted a strain on NHS resources as graduate nurses expected higher pay and were less available than diploma nurses to do rostered services.

The professional officer of Unison, Paul Chapman, also argued that an all-graduate profession was not the best way to ensure intelligent nursing practice (Chapman, 1998: 63). However, he was resigned to its inevitability. His own experience as a conference speaker to ward sisters in 1991 had demonstrated, from a show of hands in the audience, that 90 per cent of ward sisters did not think ward sisters ought to have a degree in the future. And he still had reservations. He was not against educational qualifications *per se* but he did not believe that the kind of theoretical educational courses that were attended by nurses enabled them to be competent in practice.

Chapman argued that there were no set and reinforced standards as in other professions, and educationalists and professionalizers lacked 'feet on the ground'. Clinical experience, rather than theoretical knowledge, was therefore not understood as a crucial component of competent nursing practice. In future, hands-on care would be performed by health care assistants: 'The public affection for nurses will transfer to HCAs (and other support workers because they are doing the hand-on-the-fevered-brow tasks which the public most appreciate).' Individual character was as significant as qualifications. A degree would not improve on mediocrity.

That nurses themselves did not want an academic and all-graduate profession was reflected in a survey of its readers conducted by *Nursing Times* in May 1998 and reported on in July (Vousden, 1998: 18–19). Of the 201 replies, 84 per cent thought that their profession should not be degree only. Furthermore, after pay, 29 per cent thought that recruitment problems were caused by too much emphasis on academic achievements or qualifications, including entry requirements for training.

In fact, nurses were struggling to obtain post-registration academic qualifications, which they felt pressurized to do. In the report of a study by researchers from Leeds University, entitled *Changing Patterns of Training Provision: Implications for Access and Equity,* one of the researchers,

Jenny Hewison, commented that they found 'Angels on the verge of despair'. According to Hewison, interviews with nurses demonstrated that: 'Nursing's education revolution is exerting intolerable pressure on staff as they try to juggle studying in their spare time with a full-time job' (Hewison, 1998: 14–15). The researchers (Hewison, Millar and Dowswell, 1998a: 2) found that 80 per cent of their respondents were motivated by 'negative work-related factors of some kind' and 52 per cent mentioned pressures from the wider professional environment as a reason for taking part in the post-compulsory education and training course. These staff used expressions such as 'the way nursing is going now' or 'with the changes in the NHS'. With regard to funding continuous education, health care providers argued that: 'if in future Trusts were direct purchasers of courses, then they might opt for less "education" and more job specific "training"' (Hewison, Millar and Dowswell, 1998b: 11).

It was not only nurses who questioned the direction of nursing. Those responsible for providing health care seemed increasingly concerned that current training, as validated by the nursing profession in higher educa-tion institutions, was not providing the kinds of skills needed. A briefing paper from the RCN described anecdotal concerns from employers of a 'skills gap' between registered Diploma nurses and non-registered nursing staff: 'One line of argument is that the current educational framework (specifically that for "non-medical" professionals) has fallen out of step with the needs of the health services' (RCN Employment Information and Research Unit, 1998: 10–11).

Education Purchasing Consortia (EPCs) were a strategic response to this problem. Employers (including Trusts, GPs, Social Services and the independent and voluntary sectors) were grouping into geographical consortia and planning the workforce required for local needs and buying in their own education and training. And some consortia were thinking radically about training their own staff, and hoping to negotiate with the UKCC for registration after staff had completed the appropriate courses. According to the briefing document, this would be an 'in-service route to registration' mirroring the existing situation in occupational therapy (RCN Employment Information and Research Unit, 1998: 10). But it would also be a revival of the nursing apprenticeship model, so recently rejected by the profession.

Other commentators were arguing for a change in health care that might in fact dispose of the nursing role altogether by creating a generic carer, a spectrum of roles on various levels to match workload and the competence of staff but not based on individual disciplines. This was the position expressed by the national steering group on the future of the health care workforce (Cochrane and Conroy, 1996). Moreover, while nursing was looking to graduate status and nurses were encouraged to look for promotion in specialization, such as ITU and drug and alcohol dependency, the Institute of Employment Studies (Seccombe and Smith, 1997) was arguing that the greatest need for nurses would be amongst the very elderly, the receivers of the largest expenditure per capita in the health service, and a demographically growing sector. There would be a great need for nurses in one of the least glamorous specialities where traditional clinical skills would be crucial.

Changing the nursing role

By 1999, doubts were being raised about the future existence of the nursing profession as a separate entity. Some believed that the distinction between doctors and nurses, for example, should be abandoned in favour of a unified generic grouping, with everyone entering at the same level and receiving similar basic training before branching out (Caines, 1999). This was felt to be a strategy to mitigate the crisis in recruiting nurses.

It was a view that had been increasingly suggested. Sir Terence English, a former President of the Royal College of Surgeons, argued in the *British Medical Journal* (English, 1997), that nurses should be adaptable and extend their roles into clinical specialist and nurse practitioner roles. He seemed to be reflecting a more pragmatic view about the inevitability of change. And yet he also expressed concerns. Before changes of this kind could be widely accepted there would have to be clarity about the training, status, authority, working relationships, career structure, and remuneration of those who undertook responsibilities well beyond their traditional roles. English was aware that there was worry about whether nurses would relinquish their caring role and concentrate too much on the acquisition of technical skills. He also thought there was a more cynical view – that, by promulgating the extension of the nurse's role, nurses were being used to help implement the reduction in junior doctors' hours.

The joint editorial published in the *British Medical Journal* and in *Nursing Standard* (Casey and Smith, 1997a, 1997b) welcomed nursing developments and the increasing overlap between doctors and nurses, although its supposition that nursing was now building a scientific foundation for its art seems rather misinformed. This needed further clarification, for nursing had clearly rejected the 'medical model' and with it biomedical science which, as the General Medical Council (1993) made clear, was vital for training doctors.

Richardson and Maynard (1995) had reviewed the knowledge base of doctor–nurse substitution and concluded that substitution was indeed occurring. The number of whole-time equivalent practice nurse posts had increased from around 3,000 in 1988 to over 9,000 in 1992. This had not been demonstrated to be cost effective, and the cost effectiveness of substituting nurses for doctors could not be demonstrated without measuring the quality of care and the services provided. This had not been done in the US studies of the 1970s and 1980s. Effects on patient health and well-being were not known.

Studies had shown that the higher the grades and skills of nurses, the higher the quality of care. If higher-grade degree-level nurses took over doctors' work, they themselves would be replaced by health care assistants in hospitals and primary settings: 'The substitution of cheaper (lower grade) nursing staff for more expensive staff may affect the quality of care' (Richardson and Maynard, 1995: 16). Most studies analysed were US studies from the 1970s and 1980s and it was difficult to generalize from the US to the UK, the authors admitted.

Richardson and Maynard's work focused on economic factors, but they made the point that as nurses increased in status this would lead to increases in their relative pay, with the result that, as in the US, 'unlicensed aides' would take over nursing work. In fact, 'unlicensed aides are suturing in surgeries. Aides now inject IV drugs into cardiac patients . . .' (Richardson and Maynard, 1995: 16). As in the US, so in the UK, as Thornley has shown, health care assistants – the UK equivalent of unlicensed aides – were already taking over much of what was previously nursing work.

The government White Paper on the NHS published in December 1997 (Her Majesty's Government CM 3807, 1997) approved of nurses taking over disease management but did not question nursing competence to do so. And a report by the Audit Commission published in the same month suggested that the shortage of anaesthetists could be addressed by training non-medically qualified staff performing some of the anaesthetists' functions. According to the report such 'mid-level practitioners' were common in much of Europe and the United States and were frequently called 'nurse anaesthetists', although 'they do not have to come from a nursing background' (Audit Commission, 1997: 100, para. 155). The Audit Commission also suggested that nurses could take over police surgeons' work (Audit Commission, 1998). Both the medical profession, and some nurses, expressed concern about this recommendation (*Nursing Times*, 1998d: 9).

But how competent were nurses for these newly acquired roles, now that biomedical science was marginal in nurse preparation? The example of nurse prescribing shows that many nurses were concerned about their level of competence. Nurse prescribing was introduced in England in October 1994 for community nurses at eight demonstration sites. But a study of decision-making in the course of nurse prescribing, by Luker and four colleagues (Luker, Hogg, Austin et al., 1998), found that nurses were worried about making decisions in prescribing drugs, fearful about what could go wrong. Luker et al. made light of this concern, arguing that doctors also have a professional uncertainty, and suggesting that conclusions should not be drawn because nurse prescribing was in its infancy.

The researchers, all but one nurses, and led by a nursing professor, did not examine the knowledge base of these nurse prescribers, who now had the responsibility for prescribing certain medications for patients. Neither did the person who was instrumental in setting up the project, Baroness Cumberlege, the former Conservative junior Health Minister. When interviewed after the report was published, she remained optimistically convinced of the need for nurses to prescribe. She thought experience would boost confidence. She did not give as reasons for her optimism effectiveness for patients, and she did not discuss the nature of the nurse prescriber's education and training. Furthermore, she expressed doubt about nurses' lack of confidence: 'In my many meetings with nurse prescribers I have been struck not by their lack of confidence but by their impatience to widen the scope of the formulary so that they can give a more comprehensive service to patients' (Gould, 1998: 14). Cumberlege's attitude of faith, that experience would bring competence, underlies many of the research studies examined earlier. Recognized deficits on qualifying, it is assumed, will be resolved by experience.

But McManus, Richards, Winder and Sproston (1998: 346) argued differently, from evidence in their study of medical training. Experience without training increased confidence but not competence. Nurses needed to be trained properly if they were to move into specialist practice. Although Sakra, Angus, Perrin, et al. (1999) found nurses, if trained, to be equal to or indeed, better than junior doctors – making fewer mistakes, as the editorial commenting on the report noted (Robinson and Inyang, 1999: 1319–20) – this depended on training. The nursing profession was keen to support these posts as a career progression but the academic content and extent of training varied enormously: 'There is no agreed syllabus or national accreditation for nurse-practitioner courses.'

A further example of specialist practice which also questioned the knowledge base of that practice was that of cardiac rehabilitation. A study of core professionals involved in this work (nursing and physiotherapy) found a deficit in knowledge that was not acknowledged by respondents. They did not have the requisite knowledge and, unlike the nurse prescribers, did not believe they fell short of it. Moreover, the study found that those who trained others were not adequately prepared for their role (Stokes, Thompson and Seers, 1998). This finding, like that regarding nurse prescribing, raised important questions about the competence of nurses taking on expanded and specialist roles – proposals being advocated not only by professional leaders of nursing, but also by the government, in its plans for 'nurse consultants' in areas such as cardiac rehabilitation (NHSE, 1998d; *Nursing Standard*, 1998m: 5).

A similar situation occurred in critical care. The Audit Commission (1999: 38–40, paras. 56–58) found that there was no national policy about the scope of nursing, or training of nurses, or competency assessment in critical care. A study by Goldhill, Worthington, Mulcahy and Tarling (1999) suggested that patients were dying on the wards because their need for intensive care was not recognized by staff. In fact, while the Audit Commission advocated training for critical care nurses, another study showed diversity and complexity in ENB course curricula for the current critical care courses. There was no set standard for those undertaking critical care training. The definition of competence as well as the purposes and basic elements of critical care programmes needed clarifying (Scholes, Endacott and Chellel, 1999). This reflected the confusion in nurse preparation generally, and at all levels.

An editorial in the *British Medical Journal* in March 1999 argued that evidence for the effectiveness of specialist liaison nurses was limited. An analysis of studies of nurses such as specialist nurse co-ordinators for the terminally ill, specialist nurses for patients with stroke in the community, and nurses specializing with patients leaving hospital after myocardial infarction showed variable levels of effectiveness. The authors (Hobbs and Murray, 1999: 683–84) concluded that what was most important was actual, well defined clinical practice: 'However, when nurses have a well defined role in actually delivering clinical care, additional and specialized care such as medication monitoring, or specific patient education they seem to be effective.'

The issue of competence was crucial for the new roles in patient care. A study in Bristol described a situation in which nurses took over junior doctors' hospital work. Those involved in the study were interviewed and their experiences recorded. Radical ideas in changing roles were valuable, the report concluded, but mechanisms were needed with regard to education and training, and there was a need to support the training of newly created specialist staff. Patient outcomes, however, were not considered in the study, nor was mention made of this (Dowling, Barrett and West, 1995). The question was left unanswered as to whether such role substitution was of any benefit to patients.

This was further confirmed by the report *Challenging Practice* (Doyal, Dowling and Cameron, 1998). This study analysed four nursing practitioner posts, and found they reduced doctors' workloads, but that although postholders were enthusiastic, appropriate training and education were necessary. The blurring of traditional professional barriers could lead to problems of accountability and risks of complaint and litigation.

Nursing autonomy was seen as vital to the development of the profession, and nursing development units were envisaged as having strategic importance in this objective. Thirty units set up in 1991 at a cost of £3.2 million of government money showed that the units helped nurses develop skills and network. These were evaluated in 1994, in a study funded by the Department of Health, performed largely by nurse researchers and headed jointly by a nurse researcher and a head of public health and policy (Redfern, Norman, Murrells et al., 1997). Data were collected from the nurses involved in the units and their perceptions formed the basis of the study. Data were also collected on published research projects and the perceived benefits of their publication and implementation. The researchers concluded that the units were 'trail-blazing' and innovative, but admitted that they had produced no data at all about 'effectiveness and efficiency' of this type of nursing for patients. According to the researcher: 'We lacked patient activity data. We don't know if the units were any good for patients' (*Nursing Standard*, 1998c: 9). There was no evidence to show patient care improved if nurses changed their role and became organizers of care, even though the nurses involved enjoyed the change.

While the UKCC Commission was considering basic-level nurse education the UKCC was also considering 'a higher level of practice'. The expanded role of nursing needed funding, and a UKCC council member commented: 'There is concern about these changing roles and the fitness for purpose of the people who undertake these roles' (*Nursing Standard*, 1998g: 6).

The UKCC had prepared a consultation document of its proposals for recognizing a higher level of practice within the post-registration regulatory framework (UKCC, 1998a). In itself, this document demonstrated the UKCC confusion in the light of JM Consulting's review of regulation. On the one hand the UKCC expressed its purpose of ensuring standards of clinical competence in the standards it set; on the other hand it suggested that evidence for competence at the 'higher level' would be primarily self-assessed, by written work such as portfolios and reflective accounts of the practitioner's experience. Only the proposed panel interview would counter this subjectivity. No specified or measurable standards of the knowledge and skill expected of this 'higher-level' nurse were proposed, just as they had not been at the 'basic level'.

The UKCC appeared to be in a quandary. It was trying to hold on to the freedom and flexibility of a philosophy embodied in documents such as *The Scope of Professional Practice* (UKCC, 1992b), but it was also recognizing its previous failure to regulate the profession properly since the new order, and so protect the public adequately. Indeed, in April 1999 the report of the consultation on a higher level of practice was published (UKCC, 1999b), which confirmed the confusion that existed about what constituted both higher and basic levels of practice. The report concluded by suggesting that more detailed work on definitions, standards and assessment needed to be done. The UKCC was very keen to remedy these shortcomings as quickly as possible (Skyte, 1999).

There were significant issues arising about such new nursing roles, apart from that of competence. Brian Salter, Medway Reader in Public Policy in the Centre for Health Services Studies in the University of Kent, and Neil Snee, Director of Nursing and Quality in the Medway Trust, argued that nursing's pursuit of power had been unsuccessful, whatever the UKCC's assertions to the contrary, because the courts still regarded the doctor as having ultimate responsibility. Even the nurse practitioner role was invariably defined by protocols devised and agreed by doctors (Salter and Snee, 1997). Their conclusion was that, despite the attractiveness of the concept of holistic care, the reality was that less skilled care needed to be provided at lower cost: 'Above all, nursing must escape its obsession with the seductions of higher education and the distractions of high-status professionalism and adopt a new pragmatism in its treatment of both' (Salter and Snee, 1997: 31).

The future health care workforce

The future role of the nurse had become contentious. Alan Maynard of York University's Health Economics Consortium argued for an increase in the number of nurses, not doctors. He thought that nurses could take over general practitioners' work, including anaesthesia, endoscopy, radiology and minor surgery if properly trained. In his view, that this was not happening was because of 'political cowardice in the face of doctor advocacy, which is often self-interested' (*Nursing Standard*, 1998j: 7). In contrast, Pippa Gough, then Assistant Director of Nursing Policy and Practice at the RCN, warned of the dangers of seeking professional status, now that the role of the professions was becoming subjected to critical scrutiny, and rejected the 'mini-doctor' syndrome. Her vision was of the holistic nature of nursing, and nurses 'as healers' (Gough, 1998).

The second report published by the national steering group on the future of the health care workforce (Cochrane, Conroy, Crilly and Rogers, 1999), which followed three years after the earlier report (Cochrane and Conroy, 1996), recommended three levels of worker: senior medical staff and specialists, health care practitioners, and health care attendants. Most nurses would fit into health care practitioner roles, and would fulfil a junior doctor's role. Health care attendants should account for 40 per cent of the nursing care team in the future. This was particularly relevant as that year the qualified nursing workforce had shrunk by 16,000 over the previous two years. Unregistered nurses made up 30 per cent of the workforce. In 1995 there were 96,000 health care assistants, in 1998 there were 105,290 health care assistants (*Nursing Standard*, 1999e: 5).

This second report on the future health care workforce recognized the elderly as the largest group of hospital users, who stayed in hospital longer than other groups (Cochrane et al., 1999: 10, paras. 2.20–2.24). The report developed the idea of the health care practitioner who would be responsible for the greater part of patient care in any sector. This role would encompass the current junior doctor role, the current nursing role, the role of professions allied to medicine including speech and language therapy, and the extended role of diagnostic testing. The report suggested the component competencies of the role for health care practitioners and attendants. These showed overlap. For example, the health care practitioner would perform catheterization, as would the attendant. Broadly, however, the health care practitioner was to have a more diagnostic and prescriptive responsibility, while the health care attendant was to carry out the tasks of personal hygiene as well as the observation, some assessment and planning of care.

Amongst their reasons for their proposals, the authors argued, were recruitment problems in nursing, with a minimal increase of qualified nurses and midwives of 2.7 per cent, compared to an increase of support workers of 3.2 per cent. The proportion of the workforce that was qualified had reduced from 72 per cent in 1995 to 70 per cent in 1998 (Cochrane et al., 1999: 23, para. 3.11). Specific reasons included fragmented roles and role demarcation, which meant that nurses spent too little time with patients in direct clinical care (30–36 per cent). Too much time, thought the authors, was spent on 'unproductive' activities such as co-ordination and meetings (Cochrane et al., 1999: 33, para. 4.5).

The authors of the report commented that the bursary system appeared to attract students to nursing, but warned that it was not yet known how many would go on to a non-health career (Cochrane et al., 1999: 50–51, para. 5.15). The researchers admitted that they had not reached a view about the educational academic level of the health care practitioner. They recognized the argument for degree level, which they argued was an international phenomenon, likely to be pursued in Wales and Scotland, if not in England. But they also recognized that it was unlikely that enough degree-level health care practitioners could be recruited unless there was a significant reduction in academic standards. They disputed any dilution of quality in care if the proportion of support workers increased in comparison to qualified staff. Any research that purported to show this had not examined the quality of care in relation to a trained and skilled support workforce, which was what Cochrane et al. (1999: 55, para. 5.37) proposed.

The researchers admitted that competency frameworks, on which their system depended, were as yet underdeveloped (Cochrane et al., 1999, executive summary, 23). *The Future Healthcare Workforce* was based on the argument that the distinction between 'cure' and 'care' should be diminished (Cochrane et al., 1999: 55, para. 5.38). But what seems to have been proposed was a hierarchy of value attached to tasks. The lower the workers in the hierarchy, the more basic and personal the tasks they would perform for the patient. The health care attendant would undertake many of the personal and basic caring functions previously expected of the nurse. The role of the nurse would now be more akin to that of a junior doctor. In fact, within the new titles, the title 'nurse' did not appear. Rather than diminishing the distinction between cure and care, the new system would seem to fall between both, producing workers who would not be skilled and competent in either. What was clear, however, was the assumption that personal care for patients was the lowest point in the hierarchy. Traditional nursing, in both terminology and nature, faced extinction.

Preserving the traditional nursing role

The vocational tradition and the modern world

While some nursing leaders and commentators from outside the profession were keen to make nursing into a more autonomous and independent profession, questions were being raised about the associated loss of the traditional nursing role. Raanan Gillon, for example, expressed this concern in response to Jenifer Wilson-Barnett (1986b), a nursing professor, who was unhappy with the passivity and fear of responsibility manifested by many nurses. She attributed this to lowered status, inadequate preparation and (largely) female socialization. Gillon, however, wondered if this quest for nursing professionalization and independence was necessarily beneficial for patients:

> Many of the traditional "handmaiden" tasks which nurses perform are essential for patients' welfare but do not obviously require professional status. Comforting, chatting with, holding hands with, stroking, feeding, grooming, washing, bathing, cleaning, and making beds for, other people when they are sick, are all traditional nursing tasks, and in many circumstances essential for patient care. But do they require professional skills or professional autonomy to be carried out effectively? Or is there some reason to expect that professionals are likely to reject many such tasks as inappropriate to their status and a waste of their expensive professional time and skills?
>
> (Gillon, 1986: 116)

Although Gillon was appreciative of many of the new more advanced nursing roles, he was suggesting that traditional personal patient care was still supremely important, but liable to devaluation by the nursing profession questing for 'professionhood'. His view was echoed a decade later by other doctors (Hay, 1994; Le Fanu, 1995; Horton, 1997; Gaba, 1997: 18; *Nursing Times*, 1997c; Bliss, 1998a, 1998b, 1999; Fisher, 1998: 20; Rivett, 1998; Warren and Harris, 1998; May, 1999).

Mary Bliss, a geriatrician at a London Hospital (Bliss, 1998a, 1998b) found that nurses caring for the elderly were poorly trained. Preoccupied by medico-legal documentation, worried and demoralized by guidelines, befuddled with PREP, 'mentorship' and 'preceptorship' they had 'almost given up helping patients to eat and drink and making them comfortable' (Bliss, 1998a: 152). Because nurses were now so concerned with 'rehabilitation', patients were often left up in chairs rather than being allowed into bed to rest: a form of 'torture' (Bliss, 1998a: 152).

Nurses were often 'non-nurses' who were unskilled and reluctant to do much for the patient in case they became 'pampered'. They were also not to risk back injury by lifting. They did not spend time at the bedside to give food, and did not know how ill patients were. Bliss also found inappropriate nursing of patients and nurses not recognizing signs of serious illness: 'I heard a ward sister tell a sick patient who asked for a drink of water to "wait until the domestic comes round".'

There was a 'frightening detachment of nurses and nurse training'. When Bliss approached a senior tutor from St Bartholomew's Hospital, she was shocked to be told that bedmaking was not taught by the schools anymore. It was the ward staff who were expected to teach nursing skills, but where, wondered Bliss, would they learn the skills, when even relatives were having to do more practical nursing care (Bliss, 1998b: 2).

Geoffrey Rivett, in his comprehensive and detailed analysis of the NHS over 50 years, argued that there were some positive nursing developments, such as the nurse-practitioner (Rivett, 1998: 347). But overall he was critical about what he perceived to be the loss of nursing tradition and disparagement of traditional values:

> Academic nurses disparaged the earlier pattern of apprenticeship in hospital-based nursing schools, where the accent had been on clinical knowledge of disease and basic skills, hygiene and sterile technique, and in which the safety and comfort of the patient were paramount.
>
> (Rivett, 1998: 446)

Matrons were no longer responsible for selecting students according to their motivation to be a nurse, selection was an academic responsibility (Rivett, 1998: 446). Although changes in nursing were attributable to changes in society such as increased employment opportunities and family and social pressures, Rivett concluded that: 'Nursing is not as good as it ought to be'. Once nursing had been an honourable and worthy 'job' but now its leaders sought to gain status through academia, had persuaded the government to force through Project 2000, and had surrendered personal care for sociology and psychology, practical experience for theory (Rivett, 1998: 480–81).

While some nurses developed relationships with their patients, Rivett argued, pressure sores also reappeared. Nurses, no longer starchily uniformed, looked unkempt, wards were muddled and dirty, there was confusion over who was in charge, and the personal care of patients, washing, feeding and giving tablets was relegated to care assistants: 'The nurse allegedly advocate, supporter and counsellor was replacing the nurse who comforted and made comfortable'. In some hospitals there was little oversight of ward nursing standards; a huge workforce of varying quality and professional autonomy in place of nursing hierarchy 'was risky' (Rivett, 1998: 451).

In Parliament, Hector Mackenzie, an ex-nurse and trade unionist, used his maiden speech in the House of Lords to argue against the 'power struggle' which had led to the changes in nursing. These developments 'let the public down' by replacing registered nurses with unqualified staff who were without proper training and without any statutory mechanism for protecting the public from unsafe or incompetent practitioners (Mackenzie, in House of Lords, 1999b: 41–42). Baroness McFarlane agreed with him that personal care, now increasingly being carried out by care assistants, should be part of the nurse's responsibility (McFarlane, in House of Lords, 1999b: 55).

The persistence of vocation

Arguments from Bliss, Rivett and others suggested that the reorganization of nursing, which involved the loss of its previous organizing ethic, had fundamentally affected care. Status and self-sacrificing service were to some extent incompatible, as nursing leaders realized. Significantly, evidence appeared to show that it was the traditional nursing role of care that drew people into nursing in the first place. Surveys published in the 1980s and 1990s supported this view.

Price Waterhouse argued that their survey findings showed the motivation to enter NHS nursing to be 'vocational': 'These are mainly vocational, centring on service to others, the interest of the work itself and belief in the objectives of the NHS' (Price Waterhouse, 1988: 79, para. 262). Similarly, Nessling's (1989) study of the labour market in North West Thames Regional Health Authority found that, in his survey of 7566 registered general nurses, when asked to choose the most important feature of the nurse's working life, 69 per cent thought it was vocation, as opposed to work environment (25 per cent), career (2 per cent) or pay (5 per cent). When asked to choose the second most important feature, the same survey said vocation (53 per cent), work environment (35 per cent), career (4 per cent) and pay (8 per cent). Nurses attached first and second importance to vocation as a feature of their working lives. This was also true for the motivation to enter training. Hence 55 per cent of respondents said vocation was the most important factor to affect their decision to enter nurse training in the first place, compared to 25 per cent who thought career to be most important. The second most important factor to affect this decision was also vocation (41 per cent) compared to career (24 per cent).

Lesley Mackay's account of nurses' experiences found that despite frustration and dissatisfaction nurses tended to 'soldier on, comforting themselves with the idea they have a vocation: they didn't come into the job for the money but simply to care for patients' (Mackay, 1989: 13). During her study she found that the satisfactions that nurses gained came from two sources: helping people (patients and relatives) and 'doing a good deed'. There was an awareness amongst nurses, which was sometimes made explicit, that they were doing a job others would not do. The special qualities of the nurses distinguished them from others: 'A notion of vocation is involved as well. Although I did not ask nurses about their religious beliefs, the idea of having a vocation is similar to that expressed by those in religious orders. It is perhaps not a coincidence that nuns often engage in nursing work' (Mackay, 1989: 134–35).

Later, Mackay (1998: 68–69), reflecting on her findings, suggested that the vocational motivation was important for the quality of patient care: 'Finally, I would like to argue that the idea of vocation has given a special quality to nurses and nursing work – one of putting patients first.' While she did not wish to deny the attractions of professionalizing the nursing profession, Mackay believed that 'something intrinsic to nursing practice would be lost if the vocational element were extinguished'. Mackay's findings were supported by another study (Winson, 1995), which found from a sample of 500 students that three-fifths of new student nurses expressed some sort of vocational reason for entering nursing.

The vocation was still important for ordinary nurses, much to the surprise of the editor of *Nursing Standard* which had commissioned a 'first ever survey of nurse's lifestyles'. The survey asked nurses whether 'nursing is a vocation?': 64.5 per cent answered 'yes' (Mercator, 1997: 52). 'That finding might surprise many people who believe that nursing is moving away from the notion of the profession as a "vocation"' (*Nursing Standard*, 1997a: 1). Nurses did not appear to find it inconsistent to identify nursing as both a profession and a vocation, for the study showed that 95 per cent thought nursing was a profession (Mercator, 1997: 51).

These findings were detailed to nurses in a feature article in the first edition of the journal for 1997 (Alderman, 1997: 23–27).

Even a 'postmodern' research study of nursing, published in 1999, confirmed that for many nurses interviewed the commitment to caring was vocational, although this ran counter to the nursing leadership who wanted a more professionalized approach: 'Often nurses adopted the discourses of vocation and duty that . . . many of the profession's leaders have been reluctant to accept in favour of more professionalized discourses' (Traynor, 1999: 147).

Not all studies found nurses to be vocationally motivated. A study published by Francis, Peelo and Soothill (1992) argued that there were considerable divergences in attitudes towards nursing among nurses. But while 'vocation' appeared in the title of the study – 'Vocation, career or just a job? – it does not seem to have been used as a category in the study itself, either in the questionnaire to respondents, or in the categorization of respondents into groups. This omission was likely to have affected the data obtained and hence the interpretation taken. Indeed the researchers point to the tension between vocation and professionalism. Perhaps the introduction to the revised chapter, published four years later, clarifies the authors' own approach. They argued that the dominance of the model of nursing as a vocation, with the implications of altruism and feminine, selfless care, masked the diversity that always existed. There was a 'naivety' in the 'one-explanation' account of nurses' motivation as vocational (Peelo, Francis and Soothill, 1996: 14).

Nevertheless, from the evidence there is clarity in the reason why people chose to become nurses. As Foskett and Hemsley-Brown (1998: 27) observed, it was to 'help' people. The main satisfaction qualified nurses had in their job was in its rewarding nature, as 'personal fulfilment' according to Finlayson and Nazroo (1998: 32). Despite the interpretation that Foskett and Hemsley-Brown made in their study, that 'helping' and 'caring' should be differentiated and 'caring' downplayed, this is in fact arguable. Whatever the terminology used, people entered nursing to care for other people.

But nursing leaders and some more pragmatically inclined doctors, as well as researchers such as Foskett and Hemsley-Brown, were keen to move nursing into new roles that devalued 'care', and revalued it in a 'helping' paramedical way, even as many nurses remained committed to traditional caring values. As Casey and Smith noted (1997a and 1997b), nursing was currently experiencing an intense debate about its future.

A project by the RCN (Wright, Gough and Poulton, 1998; RCN, 1998b) about the future of nursing confirmed the unhappiness of many nurses about the direction of nursing. There were very real fears expressed by many nurses about the direction in which nursing had been taken, and the loss of the caring role. The predominant view amongst the 2,000 respondents was that nursing would need to meet the needs of a steadily ageing population as well as the needs of people suffering increasingly from chronic and degenerative diseases. There was concern that the elderly were portrayed negatively in the media and in policy statements (RCN, 1998b: 3). Many respondents thought that nursing was to blame for an almost pejorative view of 'dependency'. They believed that hospitals had an important place for healing, recuperation and respite, which was now almost lost (RCN, 1998b: 6). Essentially, it was this 'caring' role for elderly and dependent people that many nurses feared was going. Respondents commented that 'real' nursing was being lost, and regretted that the public were not involved in policy developments. There was, in fact, a polarization within the profession:

> While some felt that nursing had a good track record in leading policy and practice developments, others saw nursing very much as a disempowered force, subject to the whims and actions of others. Repeatedly throughout the project, these two extreme images of nursing emerged: on the one hand the assertive, participative, positive professional able to initiate change and to ride the challenge of change from others with ease; on the other hand, the victim of circumstance, kept forever in the dark and just expected to make the best of whatever others dictate.
>
> (RCN, 1998b: 3)

According to the report these two polarities were embellished by two distinct perspectives: 'The first of these longed for the "good old days" when "caring was more important than money" and "you had time to really care for patients".' The second saw the past as largely irrelevant, with nurses determined to master and turn changes to the advantage of nursing and their patients' (RCN, 1998b: 3). Many feared that the expansion of nursing roles was undermining the heart and soul of nursing: 'The growing emphasis on specialist and technical skill was seen as risking alienating patients, who held great store by "someone to be kind, to tell me what's going on, to be on my side, to hold my hand"' (RCN, 1998b: 4).

There was believed to be a loss of attention to the value of 'core', 'essential' or 'fundamental' nursing (Wright, 1998: 21; RCN, 1998b: 4–5). There was also concern about the lack of visible ward leadership by 'executive' nurses, whose presence was not felt directly by patients and staff at clinical level (RCN, 1998b: 4). Nurses who had been prepared in the university sector said the experience 'had made them more confident, "politically and professionally aware" and more assertive'. Yet, there was concern about this form of preparation. Views persisted amongst respond-ents that students were 'good theoretically but useless practically'. Many were disturbed by the theory–practice gap of Project 2000 and thought that educators were out of touch with clinical practice (Wright, 1998; RCN, 1998b: 8). Furthermore, reflecting the findings in educational research by Tooley and Darby (1998), many respondents thought nursing research met the needs of academics rather than clinicians (RCN, 1998b: 8; Wright, 1998). Overall, many were worried by, and disagreed with, the push to graduate status, and were unconvinced about the benefits of a degree. And while some nurses were positive about nursing autonomy, others saw it as isolation, and felt that 'something was being lost from nursing' (RCN, 1998b: 5).

Grass-roots voices

Nurses writing in the nursing press and general media reflected similar concerns about the loss of traditional nursing values. In 1996, Brian Booth, at the time Associate Editor to the *Nursing Times* and a clinical nurse adviser, wondered if the academic education of Project 2000 which replaced the hands-on training apprenticeship of nurses could really equip students with the skills to care for patients. He had been 'an instant convert' to the scheme but now he thought his initial enthusiasm to be a symptom of ignorance: 'What I think we are producing now is a number of people who have been taught that, as far as nursing goes, old is bad and new is good.' Tutors, with the zeal of reformed smokers, colluded in this systematic teaching. Booth was not claiming that the apprenticeship method was superior to the new diploma system, but he did think nursing had swung between extremes, and was unbalanced. Nurses were now launched into clinical practice with a fundamental lack of knowledge, and Booth feared for the future (Booth, 1996: 57). Similar arguments were voiced by other senior nurses, who also had misgivings about the changing nursing role, its academic requirements, and its failings in preparing nurses for practical patient care (Davis, 1997; Girvin, 1998).

Howard Shelley, writing in *Nursing Times*, rejected the common assumption that nursing needed to have 'academic credibility' (Shelley, 1997: 49). He thought nurses were being dragged along the research path to satisfy an élite cadre of nurses dedicated to the pursuit of academic credibility to the exclusion of all else. Paper qualifications obtained from attending courses were all that counted. Similar criticisms were expressed in two letters in *Nursing Times* in May 1997. Jane Brignall was dismayed at the expansion of the nurse's role so that nurses were taking over more medical functions. It did not seem holistic to her for nurses to undertake electrocardiograms or intravenous cannulation. She worried that the nursing role was being reduced as nurses became medical assistants. The essence of nursing was well worth holding on to. Nurses should not become medical technicians: 'Nurses should value themselves and be proud of their vocation' (Brignall, 1997: 20).

Linda Sharp thought there was too much emphasis on qualifications. Nursing was being left to care assistants whilst 'big chiefs' were busy assessing, re-assessing and evaluating care. And for all the degrees, Sharp could see no improvement in health care: 'I am afraid that nursing is being taken over by academics whose qualifications look good on paper but are useless in practice.' And she concluded: 'Let us return to basics' (Sharp, 1997: 20).

In *Nursing Standard* (1997c: 19), a readers' panel debated whether too much emphasis was being placed on academic qualifications. Carol Singleton, a research fellow in general practice, thought that nursing needed academic credibility to prevent nurses being doctors' handmaidens; however, academic qualifications were a double-edged sword. Pursuit of qualifications rendered 'hands-on' care in second or third place.

Steve Flatt, described as a nursing consultant from Wakefield, thought that academia could not make a good and caring nurse: 'Besides it would seem that currently nurse education is a quick skim across several disciplines such as sociology, psychology and biology, with little relevance to real nursing situations.' And Stephen Weeks, a primary nurse in Leeds, thought that researchers were dependent on the hands-on care of nursing staff.

Writing in the *Guardian Education Supplement*, 'Higher Education On Campus' (Scarth, 1997: iv), Angie Scarth, a York University nursing student, was 'sick to death of nursing'. She thought that nursing was 'a dying vocation'. Orders came from a higher plane and ordinary nurses were powerless to affect major change. That is unless the nurse went into management but, as Scarth wrote: 'I became a nurse because I love caring for people – I never wanted to become a pen-pusher.' She thought that the future of nursing looked increasingly polarized. There would be a few highly trained managers overseeing poorly paid health care assistants: 'who do the bedmaking, bum-wiping, laying out of bodies and serving of meals. Some wards pressurize these untrained assistants to undertake clinical procedures for which they have no training.' She thought that the vast number of nurses leaving the profession, and the consequent shortage of nurses, was a result of nursing being now solely about 'money and management wrangles'.

Some managers seemed to share this concern. In *Nursing Standard* in November 1997, Kim Sherrington, a ward manager from Bristol, protested at the direction in which nursing leaders had taken nursing (Sherrington, 1997: 18). Academia had 'gone mad'. Humanity, care and compassion were mere 'buzz-words'. Academic qualifications counted above patient care. Older, caring nurses were alienated by the academic drift of nursing: 'The sceptic in me suggests that researchers, advisers and educational achievers prefer to talk and think patients rather than be with them.' Thinkers and talkers needed to 'get their hands dirty once in a while'. This seems to have provoked an ongoing debate.

Correspondents in a following edition of *Nursing Standard* agreed with Sherrington (Glen, 1997; Harding-Price, 1997). The debate continued. One correspondent, Yvonne Duffy (1997: 10–11), disagreed and suggested such 'dinosaur' views needed to be relegated to a museum with Nightingale. Writing in agreement, a joint letter from Day and James (1997: 11) commended Sherrington's 'common sense' view which reflected the correspondents' own sentiments 'exactly'. The following week two further letters appeared. Audrey Morris (1997), an older nurse, was unnerved by the push for degrees and felt like a 'second-class citizen' because she did not have a degree. Conversely, John Yorston (1997), Chair of the RCN Scottish Nursing Student Forum, thought the criticisms of academic nursing were 'naive' and 'insulting'.

Three further letters all agreed with Sherrington. Davison (1997) believed that experience should be acknowledged and appreciated, rather than devalued when compared to paper qualifications. Murray (1997) thought that if nursing became an all graduate profession it would need to be redefined, because duties currently performed by nurses would need to be carried out by others. And three correspondents from the West Midlands (Brookes, Bristoll and Young, 1997: 10), wrote that they had read Sherrington's article with 'pleasure and relief'. Academia was driving caring nurses away and preventing nurses building up the experience needed to acquire excellent practical skills.

A month later the issue was still being debated. Craig Earnshaw (1997: 12) from Doncaster thought that: 'Most people enter nursing because they want to care for sick people. Many people leave when they are prevented from doing so because they are busy chasing certificates.' He argued that nursing was about caring and the real issues were being lost in the pursuit of certificates.

Alongside Earnshaw's letter was another comment on the debate from James and Day (1997: 12). They also questioned the value placed on academic success and the correspondingly lower value placed on patient care. In their view the pursuit of academic qualifications did nothing to benefit patient care. Letters continued to express frustration at the academic nature of the profession and a yearning for a focus on the practical (Felix, 1998; Jenkins, 1998). For Jenkins, this frustration led her to leaving the profession after 26 years as a nurse. And another writer argued that nurses needed to rediscover their reason for entering nursing, in order to redress the problems of recruitment: 'Not all nurses require academic qualifications to provide the level of care their patients need. Who will be at the grass roots of patient care if all nurses are climbing the academic ladder?' (Purdy, 1998: 19).

Similar views were expressed more widely. In letters in the national press nurses were expressing concerns about the orientation of nurse training (F. Stott, 1998, 1999; Williamson, 1998; Gabbitass, 1998). Correspondents attributed the recruitment crisis to its academic direction. Academics had 'hijacked' nursing to make it a degree-based profession. Nurses pursued academic qualifications and this left a 'care gap' with no one to meet the personal needs of patients (Allman, 1998: 37).

A retired nurse argued that although increased pay would be welcome, it was the loss of the traditional training that lay behind the recruitment crisis: 'Making nursing a degree course means that for three years the trainees are at university instead of the bedside. Nursing has always been an apprenticeship training, and should remain so. You cannot learn tender loving care in a lecture hall, and that basically is what nursing is all about – along with the required knowledge of course. Nurses should be nurses, and not cut-price doctors' (Mills, 1998: 19).

Two letters to *The Times* believed the crisis was a result of faulty training. A correspondent's daughter had left nursing after completing a four-year nursing degree because she had no opportunity to put into practice on the wards what she had learned in her courses. She could only gain promotion by taking further courses. The correspondent concluded: 'Nursing needs practical people, and no one benefits from pretending otherwise' (Tompsett, 1998: 17).

Professor Roger Dyson, editor of *Health Manpower Management* from 1975 to 1991, suggested that the cause of the 15 per cent fall in the number of student nurses was not, as publicized by the RCN, inadequate pay, but the negative impact of Project 2000 (Dyson, 1998: 17). By switching training from the bedside to the lecture theatre the title 'nurse' was restricted to those who had gained a degree or equivalent qualification. Many of those with a deep sense of vocation dropped out, deprived of patient contact – and the profession needed to be more honest about these drop-out figures. Many others with a vocational commitment were unable to meet the academic criteria required by many nursing posts. Those who qualified under Project 2000 expected to be in charge rather than be ordinary team members, and left disillusioned – 'often blaming pay as a problem easier to articulate'.

Further letters in the *Daily Mail* (Atkinson, 1998), the *Daily Express* (King, 1998) and *The Scotsman* (Brown, 1998) echoed similar views to

Dyson, and emphasized the nurse as essentially a provider of care and comfort. One correspondent, (Harper, 1998) to *The Scotsman* wrote that her daughter, currently undertaking a nursing degree, agreed that students were unprepared for clinical care and were disillusioned: three of her fellow students had dropped out.

By 1999, regrets continued to be expressed at the loss of hospital-based apprenticeship and the failure to preserve training in personal nursing care (Munro, 1999; George, 1999; Darley, 1999). As Munro noted, nursing students were failing exams, dropping out of courses, and their eventual qualification was not preparing them for competence. George argued that the apprenticeship method, which unlike Project 2000 linked theory to clinical practice, had produced safer and more able nurses. Darley, the clinical features editor of *Nursing Times*, even wrote in support of the traditional hospital sister, a dragon who ensured high standards of care.

Similar views continued to be echoed by nurses. A nursing student at King's College, London, doing a diploma in nursing studies (adult branch) wrote in the *Nursing Times* that her diploma course did not give her the practical grounding she needed to nurse patients. As she approached the end of her training, the student felt ill prepared for life on the wards:

> Although there have been several attempts to narrow the gap between theory and practice, it remains wider than ever and there is confusion about what actually constitutes theory. In my experience, theory is dominated by social sciences and interpersonal skills. These are important aspects of nurse education, but not to the exclusion of subjects such as anatomy and physiology, pharmacology and immunology.
>
> We do not learn about when and why a patient might need a tracheostomy. Nor do we learn how the liver works or the various classifications of drugs. In short, the course is not clinically oriented.
>
> What is missing is the theory of clinical practice. Admittedly, the branch programme is better, but during the common foundation programme nursing students walk on to the wards with no more information about nursing practice than someone on a health studies course. This cannot be right. Furthermore, the lack of time to build up our nursing skills is astonishing. If more time was allocated to skills work, nursing students would feel more useful on the ward, and ultimately, more confident.
>
> (Wal, 1999: 17)

An experienced nurse voiced similar concerns. Judy Waterlow had trained in the 1950s. She argued that nursing was now in danger of producing a generation of nurses who could not actually care for patients. While she concurred with the idea of a graduate and academic 'fast stream' for nursing, she also argued that practical nursing skills should not be denigrated, neither should those nurses who chose to remain in the practical rather than the academic area (Waterlow, 1999: 30–31). Letters in *Nursing Times* in the following weeks were critical of Waterlow (Jenkinson, 1999; L. Williams, 1999; E. Stott, 1999), as wishing to return to a mythical 'golden age', although one correspondent agreed about the fragmented standards (E. Stott, 1999). But a final year nursing student expressed relief at Wal's analysis. He, too, had experienced a lack of teaching on anatomy and physiology, and felt unprepared for practice (Christie, 1999). Another correspondent was upset by her father's care in hospital: his infected surgical wound was not re-dressed for days. And the nursing staff's excuse of staff shortages was disputed by this writer: 'Project 2000, think again. We want care, not computers' (Davies, 1999).

Conclusion

Education had redefined nursing. By the 1990s the health care assistant role had expanded and the numbers of health care assistants multiplied. Nurses began to expand their roles, taking over many of the functions of doctors, although they had not received the same medical training. This policy appeared to fit with a society where altruism and caring values seemed in decline. Many nursing leaders now sought an all-graduate profession, to raise the status of the profession, although grass-roots nurses often still maintained traditional vocational values.

There were four major contradictions in the new nursing system. First, the nursing leadership might claim that personal caring was still part of the nursing role but, irrefutably, registered nurses were moving away from personal caring tasks. As the evidence shows, these were being delegated to health care assistants.

Second, the sense of vocation which still motivated many people to become nurses meant that they did not want to relinquish the personal and caring aspects of their role. But the policy of the nursing leadership was to undermine this vocational ideal and its practical commitment, and to encourage nurses to develop and extend their roles away from basic personal care. The new system therefore worked against the sense of vocation which drew people into nursing in the first place.

Third, nurses were extending their roles and taking over medical work at the same time as their education had moved them away from the medical model, biomedical training and the role that doctors once had in nurse teaching.

Fourth, the problem with recruitment, which was a motif that ran through all the debates on the future role of nursing, brought with it a dilemma. Increasing the status of the profession as an aid to recruitment, and distancing it from a basic caring role, would naturally attract people interested in status rather than basic caring. Shortages of nurses in basic caring would therefore not be addressed by increasing the status of the nurse. Basic caring tasks would remain crucial for patient care, as the next chapter will show.

CHAPTER 5

Shortage of nurses and the quality of patient care 1994–1999

Introduction

As the analysis in earlier chapters has shown, changes in nursing were designed by the nursing leadership primarily to improve the status of the profession. Although not a great problem at the time of Project 2000 implementation, it was suggested that such changes were necessary to increase recruitment and retention of nurses and reduce wastage of students. Moreover, it seems to have been assumed that if nursing status was raised then patient care would automatically benefit. In the decade after Project 2000 was implemented, these two issues – recruitment and retention, and improvements in patient care – provided important indicators to test the effectiveness of the new system that replaced the traditional apprenticeship. This chapter considers the evidence for these two aspects of nursing in the second half of the 1990s, and sets them within the context of health care more generally. The moral ethos of care, and its underlying values, have crucial relevance to both these key aspects.

Issues of recruitment and retention

Nursing shortages

As Chapter 2 has shown, at the time of the Project 2000 proposals the UKCC admitted that recruitment, retention and student wastage statistics (which were complex) did not in themselves provide any justification for change (UKCC, 1986a). Indeed, there was a low wastage rate from training courses, and the percentage of qualified staff had increased. Rather, change was argued to be justified by projected demographic statistics and a declining pool of 18-year-olds in the future. Ten years later, the question was whether the new system did actually show any improvement in recruitment and retention.

By November 1997, the *Nursing Standard* had reported that there was now a severe recruitment crisis: a decline in student applicants, a high drop-out rate, and a prediction of worsening shortages ahead. Young people were not being attracted into the profession (*Nursing Standard*, 1997d: 5). Anecdotal evidence by the RCN showed a drop-out rate of 20 per cent from nursing courses (RCN, 1997a, November 11; *The Times*, 1997: 4). Statistics confirmed the worry (Seccombe and Smith, 1997).

Further figures from Incomes Data Services Ltd (IDS) showed that trusts were finding increasing problems of recruitment and retention, particularly amongst specialist nurses. In the IDS survey (Incomes Data Services Ltd, 1997: 26) specialist skills were referred to as 'child health, mental health and care of the elderly'. That care of the elderly should be regarded as a specialism brings into question the definition of 'general' nursing care. This lack of clarity may indicate a concern with standards of general nursing care so that trusts needed to recruit people of a higher standard whom they might term to be at a 'specialist' level of knowledge and care – whatever that might be. There was also consensus amongst the trusts surveyed that the main reason for the recruitment and retention problems was a national shortage of qualified staff due to insufficient numbers being trained, although low pay and competition from the local private sector were also seen as causes.

Problems with recruitment appeared to continue. In January 1998, *Nursing Times* commented that millions of pounds were being committed by the Department of Health to a media recruitment campaign (*Nursing Times*, 1998a: 3). The Health Minister in charge of the campaign, Baroness Jay, argued that the campaign would emphasize decision-making responsibilities and seek to ditch the image of nurses as dogsbodies and 'blow away the cobwebs of old-fashioned perceptions' of nurses. Challenge was the key (*Nursing Standard*, 1998a: 5).

A survey conducted for the RCN by the Institute of Employment Studies in 1998 (Seccombe and Smith, 1998) found a further fall of 10,000 nurses on the register between 1997 and 1998, from 648,240 to 637,449. This decline was attributed to nurses retiring and low numbers of newly qualified nurses. The workforce was found to be still ageing, so that by the millennium almost half of the workforce would be over 40 years old. Between 1991 and 1998 the number of new registrants fell from 18,980 to 12,802. A quarter of nurses questioned in the study were seeking a change of job; 40 per cent would not recommend nursing as a career; and 70 per cent felt career prospects in nursing were becoming less attractive. Moreover, another study showed 42 per cent of nurses over 50 years old had left nursing, and less than one fifth of nurses over 40 who were not working said they intended to return to nursing. The average age of nurses in the NHS was 40 (Buchan, 1998).

The Royal College of Nursing expressed concern that the recruitment crisis was at its worst for 25 years. Training places remained unfilled. In 1993/4 there were 18,100 applications for 12,000 places; but in 1996/7 there were only 15,400 applications for 16,100 places (ENB, 1997c). In January 1998, ENB News reported that over the past 12 years there had been a fall in the number of students entering all areas of nursing except children's nursing (ENB News, 1998b: 6). In February 1998 the Health Secretary, Frank Dobson, was quoted in *The Times* as saying that 140,000 trained nurses were not nursing. As the cost of training for each nurse was £35,000, £4.5 billion was spent on training people who were not nursing. Moreover, said Dobson, surveys showed that pay was not a major issue (Watt, 1998).

Figures on nurse shortages were not released by March 1998 to the surprise of *Nursing Standard*, which quoted the Unison representative, Maggie Dunn. Dunn thought that 85 per cent of trusts were experiencing problems recruiting nurses at the lower post-qualification grades, D and E (*Nursing Standard*, 1998d: 5). These figures were confirmed in April, when Alan Milburn, the Health Minister, released the results of the survey of 100 trusts in English NHS regions which found that 85 per cent of trusts were experiencing problems recruiting D and E grade nurses especially in elderly care and mental health as well as health visitors (*Nursing Standard*, 1998e: 6).

From around the country, problems over nurse recruitment continued: as a 'crisis' in Birmingham (*Nursing Times*, 1998f: 7); and in Oxford (*Oxford Mail*, 5 June 1998: 1,3,8; *Oxford Times*, 12 June 1998: 1, 8). Nurses were being sought from overseas. Not only was there a decline in nursing applications for diploma places, but there was also a drop in applications for degree nurse training programmes for the autumn of 1998. The Universities and Colleges Admissions Service found that recruitment to the 'caring professions' was in decline as students looked towards more business-orientated courses (*Nursing Standard*, 1998i: 7; *Nursing Times*, 1998g: 5). Falls in student recruitment and shortages of nurses were substantiated by other statistics (ENB, 1998b; Incomes Data Services, 1998).

The Nuffield Trust, meanwhile, reviewed literature on the health of the NHS workforce, and found nurses were suffering from psychological disturbances and workload pressures which resulted in absenteeism. Student nurses were distressed because they felt uninvolved and unsupported (Williams, Michie and Pattani, 1998).

A study of the nursing labour market (Buchan, Seccombe and Smith, 1998) predicted that government efforts to end nursing shortages would fail. Student wastage figures in England – drop-outs from pre-registration diploma courses – were almost a quarter (23 per cent) from 1994 to 1995 (Buchan et al., 1998: 122, para. 8.4.5). The solution was not to recruit young people, but to encourage 'returners' (Buchan et al., 1998: 124).

By 1999 there was what was termed a 'crisis' in the NHS because of the national shortage of nurses (*Guardian*, 1999a: 1). According to an RCN survey there were 12,000 to 13,000 full-time nurse vacancies, rather than the previously stated 8,000 (RCN, 1999a). The Minister of State at the Department of Health argued that the government's advertising initiative had brought in 1,200 nurse returners, and applications to pre-registration nursing, midwifery and health visiting courses from 31,000 people (Denham, in HoC, 1999c: 1025). Of nurses in training on 31 March 1999, 6,319 were male and 44,740 were female (Hutton, in HoC, 1999d: 236).

By August 1999, there seemed to be an increasing number of applicants to nursing courses (*Nursing Times*, 1999b: 5). The Universities and Colleges Admissions Service reported a high rate of recruitment to nursing degree courses. According to *Nursing Times* (1999d: 6) that was a result of a government advertising campaign. The question would be whether these students would stay and become registered nurses. Yet despite the numbers of returners and new applicants to nursing, the recruitment and retention crisis remained. In October of that year the Royal College of Nursing spoke of 15,000 unfilled vacancies for nurses (*Independent*, 19 October 1999: 8).

The RCN evidence to the government as evidence to the Pay Review Body (Robinson, Buchan, Hayday, 1999; Gulland and O'Dowd, 1999) found that over a third of nurses would leave nursing if they could because their dissatisfaction and stress were so great. The RCN thought that the decline in numbers of student nurses might be being reversed as a result of the government recruitment campaign, but judged it too early to tell. Over half the nurses in their sample worked as staff nurses, the majority were women, and 96 per cent described themselves as white UK or Irish. Half were aged 40 or over, an increase of 5 per cent on the previous year. Nurses were highly motivated but had low morale, and many would not recommend nursing as a career (Robinson et al., 1999). By the end of the year, government figures pointed to an easing in the recruitment crisis (*Nursing Standard*, 1999f: 5).

UKCC statistics published at the end of the year indicated that the number of nurses and midwives on the register was the lowest for seven years, with more nurses leaving the register than joining (UKCC, 1999d). There was an increasing number of foreign nurses being recruited. In 1986/87 there were 37,668 admissions to the UKCC register which included 2,577 EC/non-EC admissions. In 1998/99 there were 26,934 admissions to the UK register which included 5,033 EC/non-EC admissions. The fall was 28.5 per cent, while the proportion of overseas nurses increased.

A review of NHS staffing in December 1999 (Incomes Data Services Ltd, 1999) found NHS trusts were making significant changes to the workforce by employing many more unregistered staff and reducing the number of qualified nurses. Health care assistants made up 13 per cent of the workforce in trusts covered by the survey, compared to 9 per cent in the previous year. According to the survey, four-fifths of NHS trusts reported difficulties in recruiting nurses. The survey found no evidence of an easing in recruitment and retention problems in the NHS. Qualified nurses continued to be the key shortage group.

At the foundation of the NHS, Rivett (1998: 445) argued, nurses were badly paid, worked long hours, but knew they were respected and valued. By the 1990s, they were better paid, but had less job security, were worried about litigation, 'and they had little reason to believe that anyone cared about them'. Critiques in the national press attributed the shortages of nurses to the destruction of nursing tradition, its training and ethos (Lawson, 1996, 1999; Phillips, 1999a, b; Marrin, 1999; Lilley, 1999; F. Stott, 1999; Harris, 1999; Sewell, 1999). Lilley, a former chairman of an NHS Trust, blamed élitist nurse leaders for seeking status at the expense of those who wanted to nurse out of 'a sense of vocation' (1999: 17). Nursing difficulties were 'almost entirely of nurses' own making'. This was a similar view to that expressed a few months earlier by a former personnel director of the NHS, Eric Caines. Nursing had dug itself into a hole when it lost its appealing sense of self-confidence and selfless detachment 'that characterizes nursing at its best' (Caines, 1998: 40–41).

Concern about nursing shortages was also voiced by Dame Kathleen Raven, Chief Nursing Officer at the Department of Health and Social Security from 1958 to 1972. In 1997, two years before she died, she endowed a chair of clinical nursing to be a joint position with the University of Leeds and the General Infirmary in Leeds, where she had been a matron many years before. Her worry, expressed in an article in *Nursing Standard*, was that at a time of increased need for nurses fewer were coming forward for recruitment. According to Raven, 37,000 entered the profession in 1983, while in 1998 it was expected to be 9,000 (Raven, 1997). At the very least the figures and analyses show that the radical changes to the nursing system had not improved recruitment and retention.

'Good' nursing: a question of quality care for patients

Measuring 'quality' in care

To what extent the changes in nursing had affected recruitment, wastage and questions of morale was an important issue, but equally crucial was the effect of change on the quality of care. Dame Kathleen Raven was also concerned about standards of practical nursing care. In her article, she argued that only one quarter of the 156-week course for Project 2000 provided direct patient contact. This meant that when the nurse was awarded her academic qualification she did not have the practical skills or self-confidence to deal with sick people. For this reason she had decided to establish a chair in nursing:

> to restore to the nursing profession a far stronger element than prevails today of the "caring" role of the nurse. Sick people need not only the technical expertise which the qualified nurse possesses, but also the warmth, dedication and understanding of someone who is truly concerned about the patient's total welfare, body, mind and spirit.
>
> (Raven, 1997: 26)

This definition and understanding of quality in health care articulated by Raven represented the traditional approach to quality care in nursing expressed by writers such as Evelyn Pearce (1953, and subsequent editions). It concerned technical expertise, but also 'warmth, dedication and understanding' of total patient care, the patient as a person of body, mind and spirit. This pre-eminently moral approach to quality had insisted on integrating modern science with the virtue of caring.

Because this traditional moral approach to quality was deemed irrelevant, researchers sought to find other measurable determinants. The North American work of Aiken, Smith and Lake (1994) seemed to provide pointers to quality care. This study, funded by a professional nursing body and headed by a researcher from a school of nursing, found that there was lower medicare mortality among a set of 'magnet' hospitals known for 'good nursing care'. 'Magnet hospitals' were defined as those in which registered nurses liked performing practical nursing, which were able to recruit and retain staff, and where there was competition. The nurses working in the magnet hospitals thought their main attributes were that the organizational structure of the hospital reflected the status of nursing, that nurses could practise autonomously, make decisions and have control in order to establish schemes like 'primary nursing'. Nursing autonomy was argued to improve patient care. What constituted 'good nursing care' from the patient's perspective, however, did not seem to feature.

But North American nursing had its own problems. Schisms were created between North American graduate nurses and the practical vocational nurses who actually performed the care. Elitist nursing, intellectually unable to convince health care reformers of the need for advanced nursing practice, had alienated the vocational and practical majority of nurses (Kitson, 1996). Meanwhile, North American hospitals were downsizing and laying off nurses (Clinton, 1994).

Barbara White (1998: 20–21) argues that North American nursing had been affected by a changed culture which had three effects. First, the ethos changed from service to the patient to a business culture of reducing cost and increasing productivity and profit. Second, nurses, who had previously worked under total-patient-care models of care delivery, were now forced to delegate tasks to nursing aides. Safe delegation of nursing tasks became a critical issue, and unlicensed assistive personnel were being used to replace rather than augment nursing care. Nurses were being required to work in multiple specialty areas with minimal training and experience. Third, health care was being increasingly provided away from hospitals, and there was a greater emphasis on health promotion and disease prevention.

Perhaps these problems led to the attempts within North American nursing to provide evidence for the value of registered nurses. One North American study that sought to provide such evidence found the higher the number of registered nurses, the lower the incidence of adverse occurrences in in-patient care units. But it also admitted that the evidence was contradictory (Blegen, Goode and Reed, 1998).

Indeed, a debate in *USA Today* showed a lack of consensus. One view from a Californian nurse leader (DeMoro, 1999) was that registered nurses were being replaced by unlicensed personnel with implications for patient safety. She argued that more nurses meant more skilled caregivers, better quality of care and reduced long-term health costs. The editorial view was that the number of registered nurses had actually risen between 1983 and 1998 (*USA Today*, 1999). An Institute of Medicine report from 1996 found little research to link nurse-staffing levels conclusively to hospitalized patients' outcomes. Whatever link did exist, the report said, was more likely to do with overall hospital management than simple numbers. And surveys showed that patients were satisfied with the quality of care, although there was still a lack of data on the quality of hospital care.

These same uncertainties regarding quality and skill mix were affecting British nursing. The United Kingdom seemed to follow a similar path to North America, in becoming more business-orientated with regard to health care. Management changes, market restructuring, and cost-cutting – introduced into British health care in the 1980s – began to produce an impact which undoubtedly affected the culture of British nursing (Rivett, 1998; Morgan, 1998). Were health care assistants cost-effective replacements for nurses? How would quality of care be affected? These very questions had been concerns of nurses a decade earlier when Project 2000 was being proposed (UKCC, 1996b). Project 2000 had had an 'easy ride' because it fitted in with the managerial climate of the period (Rivett, 1998: 446).

The issue of quality in health care was complex, as a British study on the impact of nursing grade on the quality and outcome of nursing care found (Carr-Hill, Dixon, Gibbs et al., 1995). What constituted 'quality' in nursing care was a wide-ranging debate which the authors had not resolved. Unlike medical intervention, nursing intervention was diffuse, and involved caring, education, maintenance, rehabilitation and support (Carr-Hill et al., 1995: 58). They attempted to measure skill and skill mix by observing nursing care and using a measurement scale (Quality of Patient Care Scale, QUALPACS). Although they reached a conclusion that 'you pay for quality care', they admitted the weaknesses of measuring quality this way (Carr-Hill et al., 1995: 57).

Whatever the difficulty in measuring its quality, in some instances there were serious shortcomings in nursing care, particularly with regard to the personal care of incapacitated patients. Often lacking were compassion and practical, physical care.

The need for compassion

The Health Service Ombudsman, William Reid, in 1995, spoke of a lack of care at the press conference to launch his annual report over complaints about the NHS (Health Service Commissioner, 1995):

> In hospitals some staff see patients as just another job. For the individual patient it is a unique occasion. There is a great deal of talk throughout the NHS of efficiency, standards and meeting patients' demands. It is terribly important for staff to remember that they are dealing with life and death. They must not become case-hardened and must remember the trauma.
>
> *(The Times*, 14 July 1995: 8)

This lack of compassion was noted elsewhere. In September 1996, the *Guardian* social services correspondent, David Brindle, reported the growing number of complaints against nurses for misconduct, including sexual harassment and assault (*Guardian*, 1996: 9). And in January 1997, *Unconditional Love?*, the Mental Health Foundation Report by Susannah Strong suggested that nurses were uncaring and without compassion (Strong, 1997).

In a speech to a conference on dying patients, Michael Buckley, the Health Service Commissioner who succeeded Sir William Reid, spoke of the series of complaints he received about the way nurses dealt with dying patients. Death was not handled sensitively, but also there was a lack of personal nursing skills and help with eating and drinking: 'Many patients had their pulse and blood pressure checked regularly but their more basic needs were often neglected' (*Nursing Times*, 1997e: 17).

Even nursing staff in hospices were affected. One nurse lecturer, at the same conference, was distressed at the way news of her father's death in a hospice was broken to her mother by hospice staff: 'This hospice was wonderfully equipped and had everything you could dream of. There was no shortage of resources, but the attitude of the staff was wrong' (*Nursing Times*, 1997e: 17).

Complaints about nursing care

The main body of complaints about nursing care made to the Health Service Commissioner from 1996 to 1997 concerned instances of poor communication, failure to prevent falls, lack of mouth care, failure to prevent pressure sores developing and a lack of training in intravenous therapy (Health Service Commissioner, 1997; House of Commons, 1998c).

Nutrition was also a problem. The Association of Community Health Councils for England and Wales (ACHC) published a document *Hungry in Hospital?* in 1997, showing evidence that patients were given inadequate nutrition and expressing concern that this was a consequence of the changing nursing role. One Community Health Council (CHC) stated: 'It seems that nursing staff no longer see it as part of their job to help feed patients', and another stated: 'Locally the CHC feels the duties of the nurse have changed, the caring part being superseded by the technical side . . .' (ACHC, 1997: 18).

The charity Age Concern produced a report entitled *The Tip of the Iceberg*, which highlighted problems and complaints with nursing care. Criticisms included inadequate nursing care and even a lack of care, a lack of respect for patients, poor communications, lack of privacy and dignity and included some serious worries about malnutrition and neglect of personal hygiene (Willcock, 1997; Bright, 1997b). This report was supported by the findings of the Health Service Commissioner and the Association of Community Health Councils.

In June 1998, Mencap published a report on the treatment of disabled people in hospitals and argued from its evidence that hospital staff, both doctors and nurses, had scant understanding of the needs of learning disabled people. Relatives could not rely on hospital staff to care for the learning disabled patient, and had to do the work of nurses themselves, attending to personal care needs. Nurses turned their backs on an epileptic child, because it was thought they did not know what to do. Nurses and doctors were either too busy, or ignorant, to care properly: 'The feelings of many carers about hospital care could be summed up as "good on the medical bit, but not on the caring bit". The NHS provides the treatment, but lets people with learning disabilities down on the quality of care.'

Levels of care were a worry for many: 'I told them how to prevent my son getting bed sores, but they ignored my advice and he came home from hospital with the first one he's had since the last time he was in hospital' (Mencap, 1998: 25, para. 2.2.4); 'David was left in a terrible state – they said hygiene wasn't a priority' (Mencap, 1998: 26, para. 2.5.1).

Concerns about adequate nutrition in hospitals, Mencap said, echoed findings similar to those expressed in the report of the Association of Community Health Councils for England and Wales (ACHC, 1997). Mencap welcomed the RCN Congress 1998 statement that good nutrition was 'a vital aspect of nursing care' (Mencap, 1998: 26, para. 2.5.1).

But whether the profession was embracing, rather than merely articulating this aspect, was a moot point, given the push for changing nursing roles away from bodily care. According to Mencap, health care professionals generally, including district nurses, seemed inadequately trained in that area (Mencap, 1998). The Mencap report voiced concerns on behalf of learning disability patients that reflected much more widely.

A UK research survey commissioned by the Carers' National Association (Henwood, 1998) found that although some respondents praised the NHS, a larger number highlighted areas of dissatisfaction with the NHS, and especially about their experiences when the person they cared for was being treated in hospital. Key themes were identified: inadequate staffing, insufficient numbers and lack of relevant skills; poor physical standards of care; lack of care or empathy; ignorance of specific needs or particular conditions; lack of interest in the care of individual patients, especially the frail and elderly (Henwood, 1998: 35, para. 6.13):

> I found my mum's dignity was non-existent in their eyes. As she was doubly incontinent they left her slumped in a chair with a pad on, but her skirt around her waist so as not to make washing for them, and no blanket, so I was making sure she was covered, especially at visiting times.
>
> (Henwood, 1998: 35, para. 6.14).

There was a lack of attention to toileting needs which often led to unnecessary catheterization. There was a lack of understanding of particular needs, and what came as a surprise, NHS staff lacking a similar level of expertise (Henwood, 1998: 36, paras. 6.15–6.16):

> My father has a swallowing problem, which I explained to nurses, and I was amazed to then see one feeding my father while he was flat on his back, his eyes shut and no teeth in! Also arguing with me that they thought it would be OK for them to give him medicine by mouth when he has a tube into his stomach for that. Lack of training and lack of listening seem to be a major problem.

(Henwood, 1998: 36, para. 6.17).
My husband was in two different hospitals in 1996. I could not believe the lack of comprehension shown by nurses and ward staff of the problems of a totally blind in-patient. No one helped him find the table, let alone the food dumped on it, and as far as finding the loo . . . These problems should be part of the training of all ward staff.

(Henwood, 1998: 36, para. 6.17)

It was not just in hospitals where there were concerns about care. In the community, carers felt they were not getting day-to-day information and support. About a third of carers had nursing needs that were not met. For example, nine out of ten carers had no advice on lifting and handling. And more than half had incurred a physical injury. A substantial number of carers did not have information about medication changes or side effects. The conclusion of the report was that NHS staff, including nurses, were failing carers (Henwood, 1998).

Evidence from a major piece of research conducted by a medical sociologist for the Royal College of Surgeons supported concerns about standards of nursing care. The evidence is significant because patients' views of nursing care were not sought by the study, but were a by-product, unexpected by the researchers (Meredith and Wood, 1997). Their study investigated the experience of surgery and surgeons and developed an audit instrument which recorded evaluations systematically and validly. The survey used closed-response and free-text sections.

The questionnaires used in the patient audit focused on the personal performance and service responsibilities of senior surgeons. Questions about the 'ward team', a general term used to describe junior doctors and nursing staff, and specialist nursing support were included, but there were no questions asking directly about ward nurses:

In spite of this, patients have chosen to add a large volume of free-text criticism of nursing care on the surgical wards surveyed. Although a few patients chose to write a praising account of the nurses, the following are representative of 144 written criticisms of nursing attitude, communication and standard of care.

(Meredith and Wood, 1997: 26)

Quoted comments followed:

Ward organisation was very poor; undertrained nursing staff; consent form was forgotten.

The surgeon and anaesthetist were first class but what has happened to nursing care? All of the nurses were polite and pleasant but very little practical

help was offered in my care after surgery. How about a nursing audit?
Not enough information was given by the staff to manage on the ward as a
new patient.

Not at all impressed with the system on the ward. I am a nurse and
standards have declined.

I felt that some nursing staff did not care that I was in a great deal of pain.
The doctor was also too busy to see me to give pain relief.

During my stay in X I did not come across one nurse who was dedicated to
caring for patients undergoing major surgery. The impression I received
was that they were doing a "job"; caring didn't come into it at all . . . Where
are all the dedicated nurses that looked after me all those years ago? Beds
not made, no offer of a drink, no chance to freshen up.

My main complaint is of the trade union attitude of nursing staff. The wards
are organised so nursing staff cater for so many beds each side of the ward.
This ends up with patients not knowing who to ask for assistance . . . to be
told by male nurses that it was not their job to supply urine bottles "out of
their sector" baffled and enraged me and led me to urinate on the floor for
comfort.

Friendly staff but total lack of professionalism. I never knew who was in
charge. Only one nurse told me what she was. Could not get any sleep from
other patients, given no after-care advice. No-one seemed to know anything
about my discharge.

The doctors were fine but nurses were the worst I have ever seen. Some
were so caught up in themselves that they never saw the needs of patients.

The night staff left a lot to be desired. The [sic] should be familiar with the
meaning of the word nurse.

In a personal communication, Meredith noted that the volume of negative
criticisms was particularly surprising to the researchers because of their
contrast with what they had expected. Patients' views of nurses in the 1960s
and 1970s, recorded in studies such as Cartwright's (1964), consist-ently
showed that patients were extremely satisfied with their nursing care. In
those days, criticisms had focused on doctors' lack of communication, and
were not directed at the nurses. Hence, it was considered by sociologists to
be of no value to ask patients about their views of nurses, because the
response was known to be so positive. The study by Meredith and Wood
(1997) seemed to turn this on its head. Now, patients were broadly satisfied
with surgeons but were dissatisfied with the nurses.

   The opinions reflected in Meredith's unsolicited data surprised him
because they directly contradicted the majority opinion ten years earlier

when, according to Bond and Thomas (1992), high levels of patient satisfaction were recorded in the majority of studies. Bond and Thomas were
referring to literature from 1987 (Jones, Leneman and Maclean, 1987) and
1988 (Huehns, 1988), when, according to Jones et al. (1987: 43), virtually
every survey contained *unsolicited* comments on the kindness and
helpfulness of nursing staff. As Jones et al. noted, overall satisfaction with
hospital in-patient care was consistently high and this was particularly true
of nursing care.

Meredith interpreted his findings as showing that patients were
confused about what the nurse was for, and what her role was. They
expected nurses to be there to support them emotionally through their
hospital experience but found them to be unavailable. Nursing had
changed and patients did not understand it any more. From the comments
raised by the patients, practical care was also very much a priority that was
not being met. Practical care, having beds made, being offered a drink,
having the chance to freshen up, being given urine bottles and pain relief,
was part of what they perceived as being 'dedicated to caring'.

Another study headed by a nurse researcher interviewed medical and
surgical patients about their experience of being nursed in hospital.
Patients praised nurses for helpfulness, gentleness, understanding, caring
and dedication. 'A few patients made less positive comments, for example
that nurses were abrupt and uncaring, but generally stressed that this was
the exception rather than the rule' (Thomas et al., 1995: 156). Patients
also made comments on instances of inattention, which the researchers
note as few in number, but which do appear to be serious in content:

> Not one nurse asked him if he needed help with any of his meals . . .
>
> (Thomas et al., 1995: 156)

With regard to availability, nurses were seen to be available, but there were
serious exceptions:

> I think, if somebody's had a stroke, they could be dead before they get
> there and find out what he wants.
>
> (Thomas et al., 1995: 157)

As the researchers commented:

> Others believed nurses did not have time to "care like they used to". Patients
> frequently suggested reasons why nurses did not always have time for them:
> these ranged from the pressure of work and "too much paperwork" to more
> derogatory comments such as nurses spending time "nattering".
>
> (Thomas et al., 1995: 157)

With regard to reassurance, the researchers noted that patients appreciated their individuality being recognized. Again there were important exceptions:

> They seemed to view the guy who had had the stroke as just a body; he was not a person at all, they just did not care and it upset me.
>
> (Thomas et al., 1995: 158)

> When I was in hospital with this very high temperature . . . I thought it was rather dreadful that my visitors had to point out that my lips . . . were extremely dry, because all I was having were sips of water.
>
> (Thomas et al., 1995: 158)

Patients were satisfied with the information they received from nurses, but the exception was very significant, again:

> They phoned my wife and said, "We have your husband, he has had a heart attack." He seemed to have no feeling and just came out with it straight away . . .
>
> (Thomas et al., 1995: 159)

Patients had positive comments about ward organization, but they also expressed negative comments about the lack of continuity, the lack of, or inadequate, communication between nurses, and confusion caused by shift changes.

And while patients liked nurses to be knowledgeable generally, and about their own condition specifically, there were examples given of nurses who lacked knowledge:

> A nurse came along with a hypodermic syringe and told my daughter that she was giving her an injection . . . she put the needle in, fortunately didn't press the plunger, and my daughter said to her, "I don't think I should be getting this because I'm having an epidural injection tomorrow morning."
>
> (Thomas et al., 1995: 160)

There appeared to be some contradictions in this study. Patients liked the way in which nurses treated all patients in an equitable manner, without favourites, but patients also enjoyed being treated as individuals by nurses, even with 'love' (Thomas et al., 1995: 158). Yet the researchers also found that some patients felt nurses had become too informal, with potentially deleterious consequences:

> They are all very friendly, and I take it that nobody is prepared to take on or

give somebody a good telling off, which I think in all well-organized
business . . . needs to be done.

(Thomas et al., 1995: 159)

The researchers described a significant number of quite serious and
problematic failings, despite what the social scientist Ray Fitzpatrick has
described as the 'normative effects' of patients who are reluctant to
express criticism of the NHS or of health professionals (Fitzpatrick, 1993).
Concerns about nursing were also voiced in a study of the management of
nursing in Gloucestershire's acute hospitals (Gloucestershire Community
Health Council, 1999).

The causes of such problems were difficult to ascertain. Research by
Higgins, Hurst and Wistow (1998; *Guardian*, 1998: 5) established that
nurses' paperwork was cutting the time for patient care. These researchers,
studying mental health, from the Leeds-based Nuffield Institute for Health,
found that whereas in the mid-1980s nurses spent 70 per cent of their time
on direct patient care, by the late 1990s they were spending 55 to 60 per
cent of their time on direct patient care. The researcher, Keith Hurst, said: 'It
would not be unkind to say that the amount of time nurses spend with their
patients is dropping around about 1 per cent a year.' The research found
also, from the patients' perspective, that patients spent only 4 per cent of
their time with ward staff. One patient is quoted: 'It can be difficult at times
to see the nurses. They're often in the office writing, or on the phone.'

Although this research was conducted in mental health the researchers
believed it reflected the general nursing situation. That this coincided with
the changes in nursing training and the associated introduction of a more
academic model of care, involving paperwork, is significant. Paperwork
was taking precedence over hands-on care, although the researchers
thought the converse should be the case (Higgins, Hurst and Wistow,
1998). Interestingly, the fact that too much administration and clerical
work was a significant cause of dissatisfaction amongst qualified nurses
was found in another study (Finlayson and Nazroo, 1998: 41).

Standards of care for elderly and infirm people

The experience of a journalist on the *Observer*, Martin Bright, whose
grandmother was in Bath Royal United Hospital after a stroke, prompted a
campaign by the newspaper. Bright (1997a: 26) wrote that his grandmother, paralyzed after a stroke, had been lying for hours in her own dried
faeces. She was lying in bed all day without anyone going near her. Her
catheter bag leaked. The nurses padded the area but refused to change the
sheets citing a waste of resources, and only agreed to do so after the family
offered to wash them themselves.

The campaign that followed led to a study for the Department of Health by the Health Advisory Service 2000 (1998). This report found that many elderly people were given poor care in hospitals. As 70 per cent of people admitted to an acute medical service were now likely to be over 65 years of age this was a serious problem (Rivett, 1998). The steering group contained a representative from the RCN, as well as a nurse involved in the RCN leadership project (RCN, 1997b), and this nursing perspective is discernible in the report and its qualifications, and perhaps contributes to a certain confusion in the analysis. This can be seen particularly in the section on education (Health Advisory Service 2000, 1998: 51), where the report noted that it was 'beyond our brief to comment on the considerable progress that has been made in the education of nurses', but then admitted that there were serious problems related to lack of skills or lack of training in care for older people. And the report argued that effective classroom education 'must include the opportunity to participate in effective *practice*'. Education needed to be more closely related to service needs. Despite the report's provisos there were many examples given of elderly patients having bodily needs neglected. Some patients were not washed or fed, and sometimes this was related to poor staff attitudes.

Importantly, from researchers' observations, patients recognized 'good' care as that which involved eye contact, a warm tone of voice, clear speech in everyday language, and a gentle touch. Although the staff may have felt rushed they did not give this impression to patients, and spent some time at the end of an interaction ensuring the patient was comfortable and had no further requests. Length of time did not appear to affect the quality of the interaction. Less good care was recognized as lack of courtesy, noisy, thoughtless behaviour by staff, lack of sensitivity and ignoring patients (Health Advisory Service 2000, 1998: 42–43). This description clearly corresponds with the moral approach to patient care that was articulated by Nightingale and the nursing tradition she inculcated. But here lies a confusion. The report recognized that the skills of delivering good quality care had less to do with the professional role or technical competence, but depended more on the attitudes of the individual person. Yet the report also argued that poor care was a consequence of training deficits and staff shortages. The important moral question, although identified, was not further explored, and therefore had no impact on the report's findings and recommendations.

Particularly interesting was a comment on the prominent complaint that patients had inadequate food and drink. The report noted that the UKCC viewed this as a nursing responsibility. But the impression of the report's authors was that while most nurses were prepared to accept this view in theory, in practice these tasks were often delegated to more junior staff, especially health care assistants, who did not have the relevant training. In fact, D and E grade nurses were taking over medical tasks for which they felt unprepared and inadequately trained (Health Advisory Service 2000, 1998: 50–51). That the theory, espoused and advocated for example by the UKCC, did not reflect what happened in clinical practice is important. *De facto* if not *de jure*, the traditional nursing role was being renegotiated and changing hands.

The Health Service Commissioner (Ombudsman): 'a lack of basic nursing care and a lack of attention to patients, their needs and their views'

In 1997 the Health Service Commissioner stated that many of the complaints to him concerned deficiencies in nursing care (Health Service Commissioner, 1997). By September 1997, the Commissioner reported a further increase of 24 per cent on the previous six months (*Nursing Times*, 1997e: 9). By 1998 complaints to the Health Service Commissioner had continued even in leading hospitals in London and Cambridge (House of Commons, 1998c; Health Service Commissioner, 1998).

The Report of the Health Service Ombudsman for 1996–1997 (House of Commons, 1998c) included the proceedings of the committee and minutes of evidence, and focused on seven cases as being of particular significance. His department dealt with only those cases that could not be resolved elsewhere; many more similar cases would never have reached him. This report was particularly important as the Health Service Commissioner was the last person to be approached in the case of a complaint, and the grievance would have passed through local channels before reaching him. There were many more complaints than those that reached his office. Indeed, as he affirmed later, he did not take up many of the complaints that did reach him (Buckley, in House of Commons Health Committee, 1999g: 220).

Many of the problems documented in the report, and discussed in the Select Committee proceedings following its publication, were attributed to two fundamental failings: 'a lack of basic nursing care and a lack of attention to patients, their needs and their views' (House of Commons, 1998c: xxxix, para. 107). Two particular cases highlighted the issues.

At University College Hospital the daughter of a man recently admitted, whose condition deteriorated, was not informed of the deterioration by nursing staff. The Ombudsman was extremely critical of the hospital for not following guidance and failing to provide proper training to staff in care of the dying and their relatives (House of Commons, 1998c: xii, paras. 13–16).

The second case occurred at Princess Alexandra NHS Trust. A 'nil by mouth' sign over a patient's bed was not observed, mouthwash was not offered to the patient, although it was available: the patient had a sore mouth, and his wife had to buy mouthwash tablets and swab his mouth herself. One day the wife visited to find her husband 'covered in faeces'. The patient died by falling from the balcony, and the wife was not informed of the cause of death (Buckley, in House of Commons, 1998c: 67, para. 486).

These complaints reflected an increasingly disturbing situation. As the report stated:

> The number of complaints made to the Health Service Ombudsman seems to rise inexorably. In 1989–90 he received 794 complaints; in 1996–97 he received 2,219, a record, and a 24 per cent increase on the previous year.
>
> (House of Commons, 1998c: vii, para. 6)

As noted earlier, the main body of complaints made against nursing care included instances of poor communication, failure to prevent falls, lack of mouth care, failure to prevent pressure sores developing and a lack of training in intravenous therapy (Health Service Commissioner, 1997; House of Commons, 1998c). But what were the causes? Were the reasons for failing nursing care just the consequence of increases in technology? In evidence given before the House of Commons Select Committee, which examined the Ombudsman's report (Health Service Commissioner, 1997), and in the consequent discussion, the problems affecting the ethos of care were highlighted.

Discussing the case at University College London Hospitals NHS Trust, the Chairman of the Select Committee, Rhodri Morgan, commented on the danger of being obsessed with 'systems, flowcharts and so on, forgetting the number one issue which is perhaps the ethos of the National Health Service'. He did not expect people involved to have the compassionate instincts of St Francis of Assisi, he said, but was astounded at the lack of 'basic humanity' in responding to the complaint (Morgan, in House of Commons, 1998c: 30–31, para.143).

The Chairman was speaking generally about the hospital, and the Ombudsman was critical of the Trust, but no mention was made about whether the training in care for the dying and their relatives was part of the training of the nurses involved, or whether it should have been. The Chairman expressed astonishment at the lack of compassion at the most basic of levels.

During the discussion of the case at Princess Alexandra Hospital NHS Trust, the Director of Nursing and Quality was asked by the Chairman whether the NHS was moving in the direction of effectiveness in high technology medical care but not in preserving standards of 'tender loving care' in nursing:

> Do you feel that the National Health Service is moving in the direction where it can get the technology of high tech medical care right much more easily than it can in maintaining the traditional standards of TLC [tender loving care] in the nursing side of the Health Service, the more general sort of attention to detail and the more general attention to those small things that make attendance in a hospital more likely to help you recover?
>
> (Morgan, in House of Commons, 1998c: 69, para. 501)

The Director admitted in reply that that was probably true, and that it should not be forgotten 'that the basic nursing skills are those that matter most to people and make the biggest difference to patients'. This was agreed with by the Chief Executive of the Trust, John Wilderspin: '. . . we still need to look at the basic standards of care and not just train staff to be high tech specialists' (Wilderspin, in House of Commons, 1998c: 69, para. 501).

Yet, as has been seen in evidence, it was basic, personal nursing care which, for all practical purposes, had now become so little regarded by leaders and policy-makers in the nursing profession, and which was increasingly being handed over to health care assistants. This was occurring even as the profession used 'double-speak' to affirm its importance.

One Member of Parliament, Fiona MacTaggart, expressed confusion at the language used in the Trust's report of the complaint. It was clouded with 'management-speak' which obscured the reason why nurses did not give the care they should have done (MacTaggart, in House of Commons, 1998c: 71–72, paras. 528–51). Moreover, MacTaggart expressed concern at what appeared to be a lack of structured supervision of nurses by senior nurses. She was confused by roles such as that of 'clinical development nurse':

> You see, there is quite a lot of people who failed here. There is the individual nurses who were giving the care, there is the manager at their ward level, there is the clinical development, whatever. Actually, in terms of the quality of care, it is a lot of people who have put up with something which is, at any level, unacceptable.
>
> (MacTaggart, in House of Commons, 1998c: 72, para. 551)

MacTaggart's point was pressed by her colleague, Melanie Johnson, who was worried '. . . if nursing staff are not taking sufficient care of patients to know that they are lying in soiled bed linen . . .' (Johnson, in House of Commons, 1998c: 75, para. 573).

Johnson was disturbed with the thought that a hospital patient could not trust his or her care, but relied on it being monitored: 'I would hope that my care was not down to somebody coming round and monitoring whether I was cared for' (Johnson, in House of Commons, 1998c: 75, para. 574). In reply, Wilderspin suggested that the hospital had tried to link closely with the training school they actually used, 'because that is obviously where these basic skills are taught' (Wilderspin, in House of Commons, 1998c: 75, para. 574). This assumption was increasingly questionable, as evidence in Chapter 3 shows.

For a third member of the Select Committee, Peter Bradley, the patient might have had better care at home. He was shocked by the lack of care of the patient, and staff who were 'uncooperative and offensive', leaving patients in their own faeces. And he thought that there was no reason to believe other patients in the ward did not have similar treatment (Bradley, in House of Commons, 1998c: 75–76, paras. 576–86).

The Chairman of the Select Committee, Rhodri Morgan, concluded the examination of this case by some devastating comments directed at Mr Wilderspin. Some very basic things had gone wrong and no amount of 'management speak gobbledegook' could account for it, or indeed, remedy the problem:

> . . . what you have put over to us is this question of developing monitoring tools and auditing tools, and so on, and yet much of that is going to come over as management speak gobbledegook by comparison with these terribly, terribly simple, basic things that seem to have gone wrong, whereby it says "nil by mouth" but he was being fed, he should have needed mouthwash as far as the nursing staff was concerned, but not only was that not done but then the patient asked, "Can I have some mouthwash" and they said. "Oh, no, no mouthwash here, you go and buy your own", and then the patient is covered in faeces, and so on. It does not matter how much you either audit or provide monitoring facil-ities, or you use the patient's charter and you routinise, and you standardise, and you auditise, and you monitorise, and all these things, but those basics should not require any of these modern management tools to get right. And it is terribly difficult for us, as a Committee, representing what you might call the interests of the general public, to accept that the introduction of all these modern management techniques is in any way relevant to the failures that took place.
>
> (Morgan, in House of Commons, 1998c: 79, para. 622)

It is evident that the members of the Select Committee, Members of Parliament, found the lack of care of patients incomprehensible. They may have been incredulous, but they also failed to understand the nursing profession, its structure, supervision and the training of nurses. They were puzzled and perplexed, unable to see the direct connection between poor standards of nursing and the changed ethos which had affected nurse training as well as ward and hospital structures.

In the examination of witnesses from the NHS Executive and Department of Health, the Chairman of the Select Committee, Rhodri Morgan, summed up the cases, and the implications that ensued from them. He reminded witnesses of the basic failures in nursing care at the Princess Alexandra Hospital NHS Trust, and hoped for some answers from those responsible for the service, so that lessons could be learned. But in response, the Deputy Chief Nursing Officer, Mrs Pat Cantrill, in evidence to the Select Committee demonstrated the janus-like position of the profession – looking both ways at once. Naturally, Mrs Cantrill sought to defend Project 2000 training, as 'the core of all that is in relation to the fundamental values of nursing, what used to be called basic nursing care'.

But her statements lacked credibility. They were deficient in both detail and content about what teaching was given to nurses in these 'fundamental values'. Merely to affirm this occurred was no guarantee that it did. In fact, it appeared that Mrs Cantrill had little idea of what did occur in nurse education, but defended herself by stating that she and the Chief Nursing Officer met with chief nurses regularly and listened carefully to practitioners (Cantrill, in House of Commons, 1998c: 133, para. 1037). The questioner, Ronnie Campbell, was unconvinced:

> Could I stop you there because still, even now with all the wonderful stuff that you do, there must be something wrong . . . You can do all the training you want, but there is something wrong somewhere . . . there must be something wrong somewhere. You can do all the training you want, but something is wrong somewhere.
>
> (Campbell, in House of Commons, 1998c: 133, para. 1038)

Three times Campbell repeated this heartfelt cry of puzzlement and exasperation: '. . . there must be something wrong somewhere'. But what was it? He just did not understand, and flailing around for answers wondered if the problem was temporary 'bank' staff, although this in itself would not have explained poor nursing care, for 'bank staff' were often ward staff doing extra shifts. As the Director of Nursing and Quality at the Princess Alexandra Hospital NHS Trust, Margaret Berry, had stated:

> . . . the "bank" nurses we use, for the larger part, about 85 per cent, are our own staff who are substantively employed working their ordinary shifts within the Trust, and extra hours are worked by the "bank" . . .
>
> (Berry, in House of Commons, 1998c: 68, para. 499)

Continuity of care was not therefore affected. And even if 'bank' nurses were hired from agencies, from outside the organization, they were still trained nurses. This is further supported by Cantrill, in her evidence to the Committee. Princess Alexandra Hospital, at the time of the complaint, was using only 20 per cent 'bank nurses' and those 'bank' nurses 'were all people who had actually worked within the hospital (Cantrill, in House of Commons, 1998c: 133, para. 1038).

In fact, in the evidence it appears that there was no consideration as to who was actually performing basic personal care at all. Whether health care assistants were involved, and who took responsibility, was not mentioned. In all the cases, much mention was made of training requirements by the nursing establishment, but they were words that did not reflect reality, or show any detailed evidence. Campbell was not happy with the answers he was given:

> I am still not quite sure. I am trying to get out of you what is going wrong at the minute because we have had independent reports from your own that the standard of nursing has fallen with the complaints we have had and Mr Langlands said before that the majority of the National Health Service is wonderful and everything is great, but we are only dealing with the cases we get and the cases we get are bad cases. As I said before, the cases now that we are getting, as I know from my experience on this Committee, are of cases where people have died as a result of bad nursing or bad medical care and that worries me a great deal because I do not want people going to hospital and dying because they did not get the care.
> (Campbell, in House of Commons, 1998c: 134, para. 1041)

Campbell gave examples of people dying from bad care. Mr Alan Langlands, Chief Executive NHS Executive, tried to paint a more positive picture by suggesting poor care was due to pressure of time on staff, and he quoted a staff nurse as saying: 'The missing commodity around here is breathing space. If only I had a little breathing space, I could do this, that and the next thing better' (Langlands, in House of Commons, 1998c: 134, para.1041). But he did not acknowledge any underlying causes for the problems.

In the proceedings of the following week, the Secretary of State for Health, Frank Dobson, answered questions from the Committee, and the issues surrounding poor standards of nursing identified by the Ombudsman in the report appeared to be glossed over. Dobson appreciated that the removal of national standards was not always beneficial (Dobson, in House of Commons, 1998c: 146, para. 1102). His concerns appeared to be to improve procedures, and he was also concerned to protect the rights of staff (Dobson, in House of Commons, 1998c: 148, para. 1115). He spoke of the organization intended to improve standards, the National Institute of Clinical Excellence, but believed the professions themselves would be responsible for setting standards (Dobson, in House of Commons, 1998c: 152, para. 1135).

The Select Committee also highlighted issues of incompetence in three further cases. Pressure sores developed in a patient in a nursing home (Morgan, in House of Commons, 1998c: 101–2, paras. 803–5). Nursing records were improperly kept and as a result it was impossible to investigate standards of care (Morgan, and Buckley, in House of Commons, 1998c: 81, para. 628). And a patient admitted with an overdose died having been incorrectly treated by a doctor, and nurses did not know what to do: 'Some of the nurses did not know what to do; they did not have a clue' (Campbell, in House of Commons, 1998c: 116, para. 916).

The cases brought to the Health Service Commissioner and the following parliamentary debate show that complaints revolved around two inextricable issues: the lack of compassion and the lack of practical care – even, and especially, basic practical care. Although the Select Committee agreed with Alan Langlands, and recognized the commitment, dedication and skills of the vast majority of people working in the National Health Service, it also realized there was no room for complacency. In the evidence given to them, they heard too many examples of poor care, poor management and inadequate administration (House of Commons, 1998: v, para. 1). As the Select Committee report stated:

> We point out that the Health Service Ombudsman regularly reports to Parliament on the worryingly low standards of care received by an increasing number of patients, and we hope that the NHS will use his reports in its efforts to improve patients' experiences of their care.
>
> (House of Commons, 1998c: xxxix, para. 109)

Difficulties in complaining

Stories of neglect in the press confirmed this. A professor of social work was upset at her father's hospital treatment: 'being dressed in ill-fitting clothes, not being able to understand the system with food, being in cramped accommodation, surrounded by other elderly people with physical and mental health problems, and above all, the pervasive smell of urine . . .' (Baldwin, 1998: 3). Silvia Rodgers' (1998: 3) hospital treatment had changed from a decade earlier: '. . . to ask for anything – water, analgesics, a bedpan – incurred displeasure. Twenty minutes was the average wait for a bedpan. Bottoms were never wiped, paper never offered. Sheets became sodden, but would not be changed till the next morning.'

Help the Aged conducted a survey of older peoples' views in January 1999 (Help the Aged, 1999a). It suggested that: 'Nurses have lost the human touch and often appear indifferent to the needs of patients.' One respondent described nurses as 'rude and offensive', another called them 'flippant'. Health care assistants were regarded as kinder and 'less callous'. Other comments noted by the survey (1999a: 3–5) raised the issues of nurses being excessively noisy at the nurses' station, not washing patients' hair, not giving patients help to keep clean, 'too many Chiefs and not enough Indians', and a male nurse looking after a female patient when a female nurse was requested and was available. Although some relatives were content with the care given, many were not. 'One person was told by a nurse that "*you are not my patient*", and so was not helped.' Nurses covered up for each other. One patient with throat cancer was denied ice that was available. According to another respondent: 'Hands-on nursing has gone these days.' There was a feeling that: 'Nurses are so highly educated, but we still need the practical nurses who can do the little simple things in life'.

In October 1999 Help The Aged reviewed its campaign activity to promote 'Dignity on the Ward' (Help the Aged, 1999b). Between November 1998 and July 1999, 1000 letters were received on the subject. Of the letters analysed, half (330) involved quality of care. The remainder concerned clinical care (146), attitude (133) and environment (58). Although Help the Aged found some improvement in the intervening years in the provision of care for older people, it also noted the difficulty there was in making complaints.

Similar criticisms were raised by a report from Age Concern (1999). Sick, frail and elderly people were left in soiled beds and without food, and even subjected to abuse. The *Daily Telegraph* (1999a) also reiterated deep and frequent concerns from the public, 'a flood of calls' about the nursing and medical care of elderly relatives in hospital. Awful neglect and lack of care had affected the grandmother of a television presenter, Liz Kershaw: 'There was blood under her finger nails. She had congealed blood around her mouth and her teeth. She was just neglected. Her mouth was full of matter' (7 December: 14–15). Other relatives reported that patients were not fed, developed pressure sores and infections. One correspondent wrote that she saw 'laughing nurses playing cards as my dying mother lay in squalor' (8 December: 4). The loss of the nursing apprenticeship training and of the traditional ward sister role were held by some writers to be partly responsible. A debate in the House of Lords (House of Lords, 1999c) revealed 60 police investigations pending on maladministration against elderly patients in NHS hospitals. Baroness Young had further anecdotal evidence of a patient 'who died of starvation' (Young, in House of Lords, 1999c: 218).

The complaints procedure was ineffective in holding the NHS to account (Help the Aged, 1999c; Wallace and Mulcahy, 1999). In evaluating the effectiveness of the NHS complaints procedure, Wallace and Mulcahy suggested that there was a fundamental inequality of power between patients and professionals (1999: 2, para. 1.6). Patients were disadvantaged. The NHS was a virtual monopoly with no alternative for those who continued to need care and could not pay for private care. Clinicians had expert knowledge with which it was difficult for patients to negotiate. Many people were not familiar with NHS workings, or what they ought to deliver. Because of vulnerability, patients were not in a good position to voice a grievance.

According to Wallace and Mulcahy (1999: 3, para. 1.7), the rapidly rising number of complaints in the NHS was often taken as an indication that users were becoming increasingly demanding and adversarial. However, they disputed this, arguing that evidence from empirical research studies demonstrated that the majority of grievances about medical services actually went unvoiced. Some users might prefer to put negative experiences behind them, or to avoid confrontation. For others, inequality in the user–provider relationship discouraged them from pursuing a grievance. Patients tended not to make formal complaints when they have to preserve a long-term relationship with a service provider. This fear was exacerbated in certain locations where a shortage of service providers existed. Wallace and Mulcahy (1999: 3, para. 1.9) argued further that only a very small minority of dissatisfied complaints ever reached the Health Service Commissioner (fewer than 2 per cent of the 399 complainants studied).

As Wallace and Mulcahy point out, complainants felt powerless, and there was an innate bias towards the whole NHS by those who were on panels of local resolution. Complainants felt that their account of events was less likely to be believed than those of the staff concerned; staff denials were taken at face value and proper investigation behind the facts was not undertaken, and investigations were superficial (1999: 14, para. 2.18; 20, para. 2.43).

Complaints which raised grave concerns about competence or conduct, and which included allegations of serious neglect in nursing care, were not considered in an impartial and robust way (Wallace and Mulcahy, 1999: 21–22, paras. 2.48–53). One complainant, for example, was concerned that the investigator had not been open about acknowledging the poor standards of care from staff within the investigator's unit, as it reflected badly on the investigator's own management abilities. Another complainant thought: 'They washed all hands of responsibility.' (Sic) Other complainants had similar experiences. In one case, the response was based on nursing statements 'which were allegedly full of inaccuracies, untruths, denials and offensive comments about the complainant'. In another case: 'One complainant who herself was a director of nursing said that the question of discipline was "simply brushed aside". She was given no assurances that the problems with the nursing staff were being addressed.'

With regard to disciplinary procedures following complaints, Wallace and Mulcahy (1999: 58, para.5.12) warned of the shift from discipline to a process based on unenforceable recommendations emphasizing retraining and improving skills. Although they agreed this could be positive, they also thought this lacked the threat of sanction and was reliant on the co-operation of the practitioner concerned. Processes needed to be made more visible.

An inquiry into two deaths at a hospital, which followed an adjournment debate in the House of Commons on 24 May 1999 (House of Commons, 1999b; NHSE South East, 1999), chaired by a regional nurse director, sought to examine the quality of nursing care and levels of staffing, as well as issues specific to the two deaths. A close analysis of the evidence shows profound concerns with nursing care (NHSE South East, 1999: Appendix (e): 1, para. 2.i). Issues raised by people meeting members of the review team at a public meeting organized by the independent Community Health Council, at 'drop-in' sessions, and in correspondence, revealed a number of criticisms of nursing care, similar to those found by the Parliamentary Ombudsman and other studies examined earlier in this chapter.

The public criticized failures of nursing care, particularly in respect to the elderly, the disabled and those with a learning disability. These related to feeding, providing adequate fluids, communicating and providing basic, personal nursing care. Many perceived unsympathetic attitudes of nursing staff, ignoring the needs of patients and concerns of relatives. In the minds of the public, the evidence for this was from staff socializing, making telephone calls and drinking tea and coffee at the nurses' station.

A major source of anxiety was the lack of regular contact between the nurse and the patient at the bedside, to reassure, observe progress and ensure patient comfort. People felt strongly that regular contact would ensure appropriate nutrition and fluids, adequate pain control, attention to personal hygiene and improved nursing care. Contact only when call bells rang, which were not always answered, or on the drugs round, did not provide proper basic nursing care for dependent patients.

Team members were also concerned about a lack of disability awareness, and evidence of nurses sleeping on duty. Other issues raised by the public (NHSE South East, 1999: Appendix (e): 1–2, para. 2.ii–iv) included poor communication; poorly managed complaints; and the need for more trained nurses and better supervision

The review team held the management to be responsible for these shortcomings by replacing registered, qualified nurses with care assistants. The team found wards to be understaffed, and believed that managers were confused about the role of the registered nurse and support staff, believing them to be interchangeable. In the team's view it was the skill mix that led to poor standards of basic, personal nursing, particularly for older, frail or disabled patients.

An admission of failing standards of nursing care by the professional body?

The UKCC was concerned about personal relationships between nurses and patients. It published research into nurse–patient relationships which showed that many nurses did not know when they had 'overstepped the mark' with patients (*Nursing Standard*, 1998b: 5). This was a feature of many of the cases before the UKCC. The UKCC was so concerned about inappropriate relationships between nurses and patients that it published news of a research project it was setting up, and quoted a UKCC professional officer, Richard Bradshaw:

> The protection of vulnerable patients and clients lies at the heart of the UKCC's role. This work is addressing a number of difficult and sensitive issues. We want to know, for example, why male nurses are much more likely than their female colleagues to appear before the UKCC's Professional Conduct Committee. We also want to know why problems deriving from inappropriate relationships seem more likely to develop in certain areas of practice and less so in other areas. Ultimately, it is the responsibility of the professionally accountable registered nurse, midwife and health visitor to ensure that at all times appropriate boundaries are maintained within the patient–practitioner relationship.
>
> (UKCC, 1998c: 9)

In June 1998, the UKCC announced that complaints to the UKCC had risen by 60 per cent in the previous year, until 31 March 1998. It argued that two-thirds had been trivial and had not withstood investigation. Nevertheless it admitted that complaints from the public were generally better thought out than those lodged by colleagues or managers. The most common complaints related to physical, sexual and verbal abuse of patients, as well as stealing from patients and failing to care for patients. The UKCC thought some of the increase was due to its own advertising of the complaints procedure to the general public (*Nursing Standard*, 1998f: 5).

In August it was announced that the number of complaints about nurses from members of the public was rising, comprising two-thirds of all complaints. The UKCC had 1,200 complaints a year and this had risen by

34 per cent over the past two years. The UKCC noted that poor standards of record keeping were also a problem, particularly abbreviations used by nurses to denote unpopular patients (*Nursing Times*, 1998h: 8). Moreover, although male nurses made up only 9 per cent of the total register, they were responsible for almost half of the misconduct cases that came before the UKCC (*Nursing Standard*, 1998k: 5). In 1999 the UKCC (1999c) issued a warning document about the prevention of abuse. Statistics showed that cases of professional misconduct involving attention to patients' basic, personal needs more than doubled between 1995 and 1998. It argued that this was because the nursing role was changing.

By 1999 the regulatory body itself under scrutiny after nearly two decades (JM Consulting, 1998a), was worried by an increased number of cases of misconduct cases involving inattention to patients' personal needs, including hygiene needs, feeding and hydration, and also other forms of abuse and neglect (*Nursing Times*, 1999f: 6; UKCC, 1999d).

The UKCC publication entitled *Practitioner–Client Relationships and the Prevention of Abuse*, was sent to all nurses, midwives and health visitors that autumn. Although in existence for almost 20 years, the UKCC seemed to consider it now necessary to 'define the standards of conduct within the practitioner–client relationship' (UKCC, 1999c: 3).

Abuse was defined as physical, psychological, verbal, sexual, financial/material, and neglect, and the UKCC was explicit in its warning. Practitioners should not cause avoidable pain and distress consequent to any of the following; verbal or non-verbal behaviour such as mocking, ignoring, coercing or threatening; humiliating, racist, sexist, blasphemous, ageist or homophobic behaviour, including sarcasm, condescension, or excessive familiarity; unwarranted sexual behaviour; inappropriate use of the client's funds; or neglect of essential care, in which was included personal hygiene, inadequate communication, or inappropriate withholding of food, fluids, medication and aids.

The document stated that people were vulnerable when their health was compromised, and there was an imbalance of power in the nurse–client [sic] relationship. What had been the basis of nursing tradition now needed a clear restatement. The patient must come first: 'Moving the focus of care away from meeting the client's needs towards meeting the practitioner's own needs is an unacceptable abuse of power' (UKCC, 1999c: 5, para. 8). By targeting this document at all practitioners the UKCC was not only recognizing a widespread need to set and reinforce standards, but was admitting to problems within the nurse–patient relationship which now needed redressing.

Quality in patient care and the relevance of the moral ethos

Causes of the problems: changing values?

It was undeniable that there were serious problems with regard to patient care and its quality. Given the difficulty of making a complaint or expressing dissatisfaction, complaints to the UKCC had to be regarded as serious indicators of problems with regard to quality. Indeed, the UKCC acknowledged at the end of 1999 that they actually needed to notify all nurses of the potentials for abuse in the nurse–client relationship. The question, however, was what caused these serious breaches in care. Inadequate care, and the bafflement it caused, may have been attributable to poor staffing levels, poor administration and increased paperwork. Help the Aged (1999a) regarded short-staffing as an important factor, as did social analysts (Williams, Soothill and Barry, 1992) and the NHS (NHSE South East, 1999).

The fact that the UKCC had to notify practitioners of the potentials for abuse in the nurse–patient relationship shows that the moral tradition presupposed by writers like Evelyn Pearce could no longer be taken for granted. Whatever the mix of shortcomings in care, it is also important, as the social analysts, Williams et al. (1992), have acknowledged, to consider whether the ethos of the 1980s had some effect on the intrinsic quality of patient care. Values were an invisible factor, marked by the general confusion about nursing, its basis, ethos and moral purpose. The vocational tradition of nursing, as shown in Chapter 1, presumed that the quality of care for patients depended on the nurse's commitment to a moral ethos towards the patient which informed her training. This involved the nurse's virtue; her training in technical and practical skill, knowledge and procedure; her supervision by the ward sister, and her induction into the values and relationships of professional etiquette. Ironically, many of the complaints, for example, those given to the NHSE South East (1999) and those uncovered by the UKCC (1999c), were directed at failures in all these specific categories.

Yet this ethos and tradition, now labelled the 'Pilgrim's Progress' view of history, had been radically overhauled from the late 1970s. Mick Carpenter, writing in 1978, argued that nurses were stereotyped into angels or tyrants or pseudo-sex objects. He rejected the 'angel image' as a form of repression of women. Only by espousing such an image, argued Carpenter (1978: 90), 'could the tender, mothering traits be appropriated and the "Gamp" label discarded'. Vocation and religiosity served not only to emphasize service to humanity, but also the asexuality of the nurse. Accordingly, the perpetuation of the 'angel' image of nurses as dedicated and serving others was now thought to be a political form of social control, 'reinforcing certain strands and beliefs in a tradition which has done little to protect or enhance the interests of the rank and file nurse' (Salvage, 1985: 33). The tradition of altruism was no longer acceptable for a modern nursing profession, even though its values clung stubbornly, difficult to erase. This had become the central motive for change:

> Today, the vocational qualities vested in the angel figure are often emphasised to nursing students as their suggested professional goal. Dedication and service to others are put alongside patience, compliance, and a refusal to be ruffled or to show feelings of anger or hurt. The "good nurse" does not complain but accepts with grace and composure everything thrown at her, and self-sacrifice is seen as a virtue – to the point where nurses are even heard to argue that raising wages would attract the wrong kind of people into nursing, and that low pay ensures getting "the right kind of girl" who works not for money but for altruism.
>
> (Salvage, 1985: 21)

A similar position was argued by Pam Smith (1992). Her study of nurses undergoing traditional training under the General Nursing Council 1977 syllabus, had found that most patients she interviewed saw nurses as having a vocation. They used words such as 'angel', 'beautiful' and 'Florence Nightingale' (1992: 30). Recruitment was still based on the concept of nurses being somehow dedicated to service: 'The idea that nursing was a vocation epitomized the belief that nurses brought not only natural skills to their chosen occupation, but also deeper qualities of giving and lack of interest in financial reward.'

Smith argued that these presumptions needed changing. She was critical of what she described as 'gender and occupational ideologies', expressed by notions of self-sacrificial service and vocation, which were inculcated into nurses from recruitment brochures through their training. Patients, Smith believed, colluded in the perpetuation of the image of the nurse as having 'natural' skills, and being vocationally motivated and dedicated; as if thinking that a good nurse was just a good woman (Smith, 1992: 32).

Smith proposed that the emotional components of caring required formal and systematic training in order to manage feelings. This required a theoretical base such as psychology, sociology and the acquisition of complex interpersonal skills, as well as conceptually developed nursing theories: 'In this way emotion work will be made visible and valued in its own right and not viewed as *just* part of the package of women's work' (Smith, 1992: 139).

The new ethos of nursing was underpinned by this kind of critical thinking and argumentation. It was no longer acceptable for nurses to consider themselves as vocationally motivated, or indeed, for patients to have these expectations. Quality care was now to depend on the acquisition of complex skills which would increase the marketable value of the individual professional, and of the profession generally. Indeed, at the start of the year 2000, *Nursing Times* (2000a: 16) commented that it was encouraging that, in its view, 'nursing has ditched the idea that the profession is a vocation'. The critique of vocation was ongoing and pervasive (Hallam, 2000).

Two questions follow from this approach which nursing now developed. First, in a cost-driven and cost-conscious market, would the argument be accepted that basic and personal nursing care required a complex and expensive educational system, when it would appear that washing, clearing away excreta and helping people eat, could be done by anyone, with minimal training and at lower cost? Second, without a strong service ethic and ethos would people still choose to perform such tasks for love rather than money? These two questions bring into focus the relationship between the destruction of the values of vocation, the low morale of nursing, qualified nursing shortages, and weaknesses in patient care at the most personal level.

Shifting values: from a vocational calling to a professional technique?

The first issue is the cultural shift which involved different values, described by Katherine Williams (1978) as 'ideologies'. She has argued that the vocational ideology was particularly relevant to conditions of helplessness in Victorian society. To deal with washing, feeding and cleaning away excretions, 'physically repugnant to both nurse and patient', if dealt with as a sacrificial act, retrieved the status of the nurse performing the tasks, as well as for the person for whom the tasks were performed, for 'to be "called" to such work, to perform it sacrificially, is to sanctify and consecrate both task and person':

> The adult status of the sick person is retrieved through the fact that any task performed for him is regarded by the nurse as her privilege, for through it she finds the satisfaction and fulfilment of her calling. The sick person's worth is thus restored through an evaluation of him that transcends the normal and more secular definitions of adulthood.
>
> (Williams, 1978: 40)

Williams first prepared this paper in 1972, and refers to RCN evidence (RCN, 1971) submitted to the Briggs Committee (Report of the Committee on Nursing, 1972) to underpin the conception of professional ideology with which she draws her contrast. With professional ideology, she argued, the nurse performs tasks that are highly skilled, concentrating on techniques, skilled judgement and action. The focus on the patient as a helpless human being is readjusted, and redefined 'through the emphasized use of clinical terms and clinically oriented judgements and behaviours of the nurse' (Williams, 1978: 42). The professional 'ideology' to which Williams refers, was merely an aspiration of some nursing leaders, and had not filtered into the profession.

As MacGuire (1961) has shown, vocational values were central during that period, although Smith (1992: 32), writing at the point of the shift, denies this. Certainly, it was not just low pay that was the cause of nurses leaving the profession. A questionnaire survey in the mid-1980s that asked nurse leavers why they left nursing found that their two main reasons for joining the profession initially were the 'opportunity to work with people' (64 per cent) and 'to be part of a caring team' (63 per cent) (Williams, Soothill, Barry, 1992: 221). The reason why these nurses left their jobs, as responses from the questionnaires and supplementary interviews showed, was that they no longer felt they were part of a caring team, nor were they able to offer what the patients needed and wanted.

As the researchers emphasized, pay was not a primary issue, neither was it the nursing work itself. It was the working conditions that were the main source of discontent. Indeed, the researchers noted that the criticisms nurse leavers had were not with matters that are an inherent part of the job, like bedpans, faeces and vomit: 'Nurses seem to accept these unalterable facts of human frailty' (Williams et al., 1992: 221). The authors attributed the cause of discontent to the growing individualism of the period: '. . . the individualistic philosophy so enthusiastically encouraged during the 1980s is totally disruptive in operation on the wards'. And they quote one respondent as exemplifying this conclusion:

> It was really happy and we had a real good team. That's what's missing, a team; everyones individuals on a ward now, we're not part of a team . . . there's no loyalty. I mean they haven't even got loyalty to each other, so how can they have loyalty to team . . . so it's dog eat dog, a matter of survival. [sic]
>
> (Williams et al., 1992: 222)

The researchers may have had in mind the individualistic management philosophy and culture of health care during this period. Nevertheless, this same philosophy had obtruded into nursing. Instead of an ethos in which nurses were a key part of a moral, altruistic community of service, the philosophy underpinning nursing was now individualistic. The regulatory body and nursing leaders, in line with current thinking, had elevated professional autonomy, and correspondingly undermined the ideals of vocational service. The very basic elements of care – washing and feeding patients, attending to toilet needs – seemed to be affected by the new ethos. These apparently simple tasks were traditionally the key responsibilities of nurses, as the nurses interviewed by Williams et al. (1992) expected.

But as nursing became increasingly professionalized over this period, these key tasks were gradually being undertaken by non-nurses. The culture of nursing had changed. And it is more than likely that nurses entering nursing for vocational reasons were discouraged from altruism and encouraged to place their practice and motivation upon professionalized values. This was certainly the finding of Fred Davis (1975) with regard to North American nurses and their process of socialization, and it may be a similar process that led Smith to conclude from her interviews that: 'Students vigorously reject the view that they are vocationally motivated to become nurses' (Smith, 1992: 32).

The parallels with North American nursing seem inescapable. Fred Katz, writing in 1969, observed that the rank and file North American nurses were not as keen as their leaders on this process of professionalization. They were satisfied to be practising nurses without too much responsibility (Katz, 1969: 73). Nurses interviewed by Katz told him that at the heart of being a professional nurse was a commitment to personal care of patients, not a commitment to abstract systems of knowledge (Katz, 1969: 76). This echoed British nursing at that period, as seen in Chapter 1.

Personal nursing care: a marketable commodity?

The second question relates to the market, and the commodification of caring. As Dingwall and McIntosh point out, writing in 1978, the relegation of basic, personal nursing care to less skilled personnel – a consequence of narrow economic rationality, problems of retention and recruitment, as well as a changed ethos – could have profound consequences for those patients needing basic care alone. As evidence they cite a paper by Stannard (1978). He found from his research in North America that many employees in a nursing home tended to occupy marginal positions in the labour market. This contributed to their poor, even abusive, treatment of the elderly people in their care. The question that arises from this analysis is whether material rewards and increased status can provide the incentive to be the driving force of care, rather than a reliance on altruism and sacrificial service. This crucial question marks the dichotomy between traditional and modern nursing perspectives.

With the shift of motivating values comes a subtle shift of purpose. With the vocational model of nursing the focus is the patient, and service to the patient is the end in itself. With the professional model, this purpose is much less direct. Although the purpose is still avowed as service to the patient, in reality it is clouded by professional self-interest. At the simplest level, the nursing professional, to be worthy of material reward, must have a knowledge and skill base of specific, competitive, marketable value, beyond the simple and basic practicalities of personal care. Hence, the nursing professional is encouraged to concentrate on technique and complexity, and to relegate apparently simple and uncomplicated tasks of care to the health care assistant. The personal care of the patient, which required, above all, a practical moral ethos, is thereby devalued in market terms, materially and in terms of status, by the health care system. Consequentially, those who perform personal care are regarded as having lower marketable worth. As Katz (1969: 67) has observed, 'tender loving care' – the essence of this form of intimate personal care – is a non-negotiable currency of temporary pleasant feelings: it does not involve social recognition in the form of a respectable wage.

The tradition, however, never saw such a dichotomy. From the traditional vocational perspective, the science and art of nursing were applied to 'total patient care'. It presumed the inextricable mixture of complex technology and simple moral practicality, directed at the needs of the patient as a whole person. Science advanced, and was applied to patients, but the needs of the patient did not change. The technical and the personal were not separable. Moreover, while attending to the intimacies of personal care the nurse could observe the patient's condition, and, indeed, build the relationship of trust and understanding that was central. Such personal care was no easy, less-skilled option. It was just as valuable as biomedical technique, involving a very complex induction of the nurse into sensitivity, compassion, gentleness, deft touch and practical skill and knowledge needed for safe and kind performance. An art, to be learned like an art, because it did not come naturally.

The consequences of the loss of nursing tradition: a crisis in nursing?

The move towards nursing autonomy, a 'freedom to practise', had rejected the stereotyped hallmarks of nursing tradition, as rigid ward routines. The result was that formality in relationships, authority, discipline and respect, and deference towards the ward sister and the doctor all disappeared. The work of Isabel Menzies (1970) on nursing anxiety was often cited as a seminal influence on these changes stemming from such typologies (for example, Binnie and Titchen, 1999: 11).

Ironically, however, Isabel Menzies (now Menzies-Lyth) came to lament the loss of the traditional nursing approach 40 years later. Menzies-Lyth (1999: 207) did not find nursing practice to have improved during that period. On the contrary, she argued that there was now a multi-faceted crisis in patient care: 'The increase in serious complaints about nursing care is only the "tip of the iceberg".' There were smaller but distressing failures now rife. What the ward sister had previously controlled – boundary control, control of comings-and-goings, and the management of visitors – was now gone. Menzies-Lyth noted erotic and lewd behaviour. Nurses were frustrated and disappointed.

For her part, she attributed this to the rise of the managerial culture in nursing, and the disappearance of the ward sister, who had managed all the staff who worked on her ward, including nurses, orderlies and cleaners. Forty years earlier she had given a paper to a group of Health Service professionals, who were heads of units:

> I began by saying "I am going to address you today as managers". That opening evoked a wave of outrage. The audience thought of themselves as caring professionals and dissociated themselves from managers who, in their fantasies, were ruthless, inhuman and authoritarian. Such a remark would not provoke outrage today. Being a manager is commonly explicit, and consciously accepted.
>
> (Menzies-Lyth, 1999: 207)

Now, wrote Menzies-Lyth, ward sisters were confused about their roles, and even a Professor of Nursing had no authority over students on placement. This had serious consequences for patient care, including the current concerns over poor nutrition. Menzies-Lyth suggested that part of the problem was the failure to clarify the new roles and functions that had developed, and the failure to differentiate between 'authority' and 'authoritative'. The loss of the ward sister role and the authority vested in it was a direct consequence of the preoccupation with autonomy. Hence, according to Menzies-Lyth, the ward sister was often undeservedly reputed to be harsh and authoritarian. Now the balance had swung too far:

> The swing has been too great once more, and managers are not authoritative enough. They fail to operate with appropriate firmness. There is too much *laissez-faire*, and "do your own thing". In consequence management is poor and ineffectual, which is bad for morale, since people feel unsupported and insecure.
>
> (Menzies-Lyth, 1999: 212)

In the same journal in which Menzies-Lyth wrote, *Psychoanalytic Psychotherapy*, a nurse who had trained 30 years previously also wrote on the crisis in nursing. Fabricius argued that nursing had lost its self-esteem. This was self-inflicted, because it had 'sold out on its essentials . . . the willingness and capacity to think about people who are suffering in order to give proper consideration to their problems and appropriate ways of helping' (Fabricius, 1999: 204). Nursing now saw itself as second class in comparison to medicine, physically and psychologically menial. The technical and intellectual were idealized and 'real nursing' was denigrated (Fabricius, 1999: 205). Academic study in subjects such as science and literature might have their uses in nursing, Fabricius suggested, but questing purely for academic acceptance in order to raise the status of nursing was to deny the core reality of nursing.

These writers affirmed what was being stated by other commentators, such as Geoffrey Rivett (1998) and Mary Bliss (1999). The nurse had become 'lost', experiencing anomie and alienation, disorientated and uprooted from the reality of patient care and the skills needed. She was now in a state of contradiction. The key question at the heart of this analysis seems to be whether there may be some causal link between the professionalization of nursing, the marginalization of the vocational ethic of sacrificial service, and the haphazard quality of basic and personal nursing care for patients that was occurring at the end of the twentieth century.

This same issue has been debated by social policy analysts with regard to motivation. For Richard Titmuss (1970), altruism was fundamental to public service. More recently, Julian Le Grand (1997) developed a metaphor by which he characterized people motivated by altruism as 'knights', as opposed to those motivated by self-interest, whom he termed 'knaves'. Le Grand himself was agnostic about human motivation, and sought a pragmatic middle way that did not depend on either motivation. But Richard Titmuss's (1970) argument on behalf of altruism appears extremely applicable to nursing. As he argued, the organization and structure of social organizations can foster or discourage altruism. In relation to nursing, the question is whether, according to Titmuss's analysis, professionalization had affected altruism. And indeed, whether the optimistic assumption was justified that basic nursing caring was just 'there' and did not need reinvigorating during training.

Conclusion

The last decade of the twentieth century saw crises in recruitment and retention of registered nurses. Student applications declined, although there was some reversal after the government advertising campaign. The drop-out rate from courses was high. Registered nurses were leaving the profession, morale was low. There was a 28.5 per cent fall in the number of registrations to the UKCC register in 1998/99 compared to 1986/7, when Project 2000 was being proposed. The number of nurses on the UKCC register was the lowest for seven years, and more nurses were leaving than joining. Of this number of new registrations, the proportion of nurses from overseas had also increased.

These statistics directly contradicted a key aspiration of the new educational programme, Project 2000, to increase recruitment and retention in the following decade. The last decade of the twentieth century also brought criticisms of the quality of personal nursing care, particularly for the old, frail and vulnerable. These patients were not a minority. People aged over 65 – the elderly – now made up 70 per cent of all acute medical admissions to hospital. Serious concerns were raised about what had once been the essential purpose of nursing – compassionate care of the human person. The effectiveness of Project 2000, as the year 2000 was reached, was called into serious question by these two key issues: shortages of nurses, and inadequate personal care of patients.

Changes in values had radically affected recruitment and retention of nurses and also the intrinsic quality of patient care, if only as one among several causes. Project 2000 had coincided with the introduction of a market-driven culture in the NHS, bringing problems similar to those found within North American 'managed care', about skill-mix, the nature of quality, and the motivation of nurses to care. Nursing had changed from what was primarily a paid vocational service to a status-conscious profession dependent on higher material rewards and benefits. The consequence was a dualism: nursing care that was highly valued because it was high status and therefore highly rewarded economically, and nursing care that was considered menial and lower value, and with lower economic rewards. The direction of the nursing profession was increasingly unclear, as the next chapter will show.

CHAPTER 6

Parliamentary reaction to Project 2000 and the nursing system 1990–2000

Introduction

The government had agreed to the introduction of Project 2000 because it trusted the leadership of the profession, and assurances of self-regulation. Although some concerns were raised by, for example, John Moore, Secretary of State for Health during the mid-1980s, about replacement for student nurses on the wards, there was a general feeling amongst many politicians that the professions could be trusted to monitor their own standards. The period from 1991 to 2000 brought a questioning of this approach, as politicians of all parties saw the impact of nursing policy changes in clinical practice. This chapter will focus on the gathering of parliamentary evidence, and chart the anxieties such evidence gradually generated in the minds of MPs and members of the House of Lords.

The government reaction to change 1991–1992

House of Lords debate

As recorded in Hansard, changes in nursing continued to be approved by Parliament in the early 1990s, although questions were gradually being raised. In 1991 the House of Lords debated a Nurses, Midwives and Health Visitors Bill dealing with details of the UKCC and its composition. Two-thirds were to be elected and one-third appointed by the Secretary of State. The Bill also dealt with appointments to the National Boards. No account was taken of Lord Smith's concerns, expressed in 1979, about representation on the Council from the medical profession.

Baroness McFarlane acknowledged the increased sophistication in medical care and argued a commensurate need for sophistication in nursing care. Increasing numbers of specialities, including oncology, palliative care, special care baby units and health visitor stress counselling clinics, needed nurses who were adequately prepared and regulated (McFarlane, in HoL, 1991a: 494–95).

Baroness Cumberlege, a minister in the Conservative government and a member of the UKCC since 1988 with experience of professional conduct committees, supported the changes: 'I support them in their struggle to shake off the image of being angels or handmaidens. We know that they constitute a large, highly trained and scrupulously monitored professional body.' She agreed with McFarlane about the level of nursing skill and high degree of sophistication needed in the technological age. But, along with the professions and the UKCC itself, she urged that good quality care embraced not only technological skills but also compassion, gentleness and respect for one another: 'British nursing in my view succeeds in maintaining that very difficult balance.'

Cumberlege wished to advance the role of the nurse into increased autonomy and independence. Macmillan nurses and terminal care sisters were the experts in caring for the dying but they were not credited with the sense and skill to vary pain-relieving drugs. She was strongly committed to bringing in nurse-prescribing, and wanted nurses to take over some medical functions. To this end she cited a poll and from it argued that many people who needed medical attention did not want or need to see a doctor but would prefer to see a nurse. Seeing a doctor was not always best for patients, and anyway many GPs were overworked and would appreciate relief by nurse practitioners. Cumberlege was optimistic that nurses could extend their roles in this way but did not suggest any means by which these quasi-medical roles would be produced or assured (Cumberlege, in HoL, 1991a: 496–97).

Baroness Cox, a former nurse, argued that the proposed Bill was to provide for effective professional self-regulation based on the principles of professional responsibility and accountability. Project 2000 was designed to give student nurses professional education rather than basic training; to enable them to understand the theory underpinning practice; and to think through the assumptions and implications of their professional responsi-bilities. This contrasted with her own training. Her first ward report was from a 'marvellous' ward sister whom she admired to that day. But, after giving Cox a good report, she offered her a kindly word of advice: 'In your own interests, nurse, as you go through the hospital, please do not ask so many awkward questions' (Cox, in HoL, 1991a: 498–99).

Cox agreed with McFarlane that complex professional practice involved clinical, ethical, legal and social aspects of care and needed a better educated and more ethically aware practitioner. As Chairman of the Health Studies Committee of the Council for National Academic Awards, Cox had undertaken joint validations of new courses with National Board colleagues and she commended their high standard of work. Validation visits were often arduous and challenging, complex and serious (Cox, in HoL, 1991a: 499). But Cox makes no mention in this speech of her concerns, expressed elsewhere, about the 'abreaction' from the medical model and associated issues over clinical competence (Cox, 1993).

Several Lords admitted their own ignorance of the nursing profession. Lord Meston, legal assessor of the UKCC, congratulated that body for its efficiency and high standards; although he also admitted in his speech that he did not 'properly understand' areas of the profession. His perspective was limited and the UKCC knew well its own business (Meston, in HoL, 1991a: 501). Lord Auckland's knowledge of nursing came through his daughter, a practice nurse, and he agreed with Cumberlege that such nurses needed more responsibility (Auckland, in HoL, 1991a: 504). Baroness Hooper summed up: this Bill marked a milestone in the history of nursing, the coming of age of the profession (Hooper, in HoL, 1991a: 507).

Concerns were, however, expressed that the nursing boards should not become over-academic but reflect and represent grass-roots experience: 'We want to ensure that teachers rather than theorists, people with experience of teaching nursing, midwifery and health visiting, are specified' (Carter, in HoL, 1991b: 1284). Boards needed people who had down-to-earth experience of teaching nursing, rather than those experienced in general education (McFarlane of Llandaff, in HoL, 1991b: 1284–85). According to Baroness Cumberlege on behalf of the government, the government had invested £100 million per year on nurses' bursaries. On top of this were the costs to colleges as well as nurse tutors' costs: 'As a nation we have invested large sums in the training not only of nurses but more recently of health care assistants' (Cumberlege, in HoL, 1991b: 1291–92). Cumberlege acknowledged the growth in numbers of health care assistants; presumably to replace the supernumerary student nurses, a key requirement to the government's acceptance of the Project 2000 proposals in 1988 (Moore, 1988).

The Lords understood the significance of education and training on the quality of patient care. As Baroness Hooper, the government minister, stated: 'We take education and training very seriously since it affects the quality of care of patients, which at the end of the day is what the National Health Service is all about.' The government had a duty to ensure an adequate supply of properly trained nurses, midwives and health visitors. Post-registration training was expected to cover general in-service skills such as information technology and management, but also the development of specific professional skills (Hooper, in HoL, 1991b: 1293–94). New methods of training nurses were now well established. There was even potential for nurse training to be totally removed from the health service and moved under the auspices of the Department of Education (Baroness Robson of Kiddington, in HoL, 1991b: 1295).

In all of this the government had been advised by the UKCC, and was impressed by the precision and quality of the advice given by its Registrar, Mr Colin Ralph (Baroness Cumberlege, in HoL, 1991c: 529). Ralph (1993: 58–61) was personally a firm believer in self-regulation. He saw this as a contract between the profession and the public, which involved the provision of safe and skilled care of a selfless kind: 'with a concentration on meeting the needs of patients and not on any one overriding gain for the nurse'. But he also wrote of self-regulation as the means of empowering the profession by enabling it to have a high degree of control and influence. To move out of the dark and into the light was a 'complex step that requires a high degree of organization and tactical skill on the part of key nursing leaders supported by their professional colleagues'.

By November 1994, Colin Ralph had resigned from this position, following seven months of disquiet and an investigation over the appointment of a close friend to a senior position and an oppressive management style (*Nursing Times*, 1994: 5; Carlisle, 1994: 16). This resignation followed a perception that the UKCC was shrouded in secrecy, a concern that Ralph had strongly denied (Ogden, 1993). Trust was at the heart of professional self-regulation. But could the professions be trusted to regulate themselves without succumbing to other, more mixed motives of professionalization, that is as a means of gaining control and asserting influence, as Ralph had described? This question formed part of the debate that followed.

House of Commons debate

In the House of Commons, the Secretary of State for Health, Virginia Bottomley, affirmed that the principle of professional self-regulation for the three professions, established in the 1979 Act, was to be further developed in the Bill. Since the establishment of Project 2000, £207 million had been spent on the new form of nurse training. In 1991–92, £770 million was spent on pre- and post-registration training, and in 1992–93, £870 million would be spent. She also asserted that wastage rates in the health service over these years had never been lower (Bottomley, in HoC, 1992a: 697–703). The debate that followed provides insight into important differences of approach with regard to nursing.

Sylvia Heal emphasized that nursing preparation should take account of developments such as nurse-prescribing and nurse-practitioners, and offer training in bereavement and other counselling skills, as well as improvement of inter-personal skills generally (Heal, in HoC, 1992a: 703–7). Roger Sims expressed his appreciation at the diligence and sympathetic care of nurses which he had recently experienced, and believed that British nurses were in demand in other countries because of their high standard of education and professional performance. But, as a lay member of the General Medical Council, he was anxious that there should be non-professional representation on the UKCC. Patients, as users of nurses' services, should have a voice on the Council (Sims in HoC, 1992a: 708–9).

Gwyneth Dunwoody did not, however, share Sims' optimism. She was concerned about the effects of change. In the first wave of trusts, the word 'nursing' seemed to have disappeared from job descriptions – there were hardly any senior nursing posts listed in the trusts, which boded ill for proper representation at every level of the professional structure. In the preceding seven months she had had a close association with the health service as a patient, as the grandmother of a patient and as the daughter of a patient and with a large number of London teaching hospitals: 'It is about time that the House of Commons realized that there is no point in bringing forward structures in which we talk about a high level of nursing care if, when it comes to the point, there is nobody on the wards capable of carrying out that level of nursing.' It should be a matter of concern if a nurse appeared at the beginning of the shift saying, 'My name is Susan, and I am looking after you,' and was never seen again because she was an agency nurse who like many others was brought in large numbers, knew no one on the ward and was unable to have a relationship with the patients (Dunwoody, in HoC, 1992a: 714–15).

Virginia Bottomley was keen to emphasize the self-regulatory nature of the Bill, and accordingly cautioned against a bureaucratic and prescriptive approach tying the UKCC's hands. She also drew attention to the particular professional skills, autonomy and individual judgement of community nurses (Bottomley, in HoC, 1992a: 721–22). Total trust was placed in the professional body by the government.

At the meeting of the Standing Committee which debated the Bill, the issue of lay representation was again raised by Sims (Sims, in HoC, 1992b: 13). Ann Winterton supported the argument for the common sense input of lay representation and the need for a more patient-sensitive service. She pointed to the danger that professions were inclined to be 'incestuous' (Winterton, in HoC, 1992b: 14). In response, Bottomley maintained her confidence in the profession to regulate itself. She did not want to be prescriptive but to maintain flexibility: 'My view remains that it would be wrong for us now to prescribe precisely what arrangements should be set in a legislative framework and tie the hands of the UKCC . . . We believe that we have found the most flexible and effective way of ensuring that minority interests are represented. An element of flexibility is built in . . .' (Bottomley, in HoC, 1992b: 20–22).

Tom Pendry stressed the importance of practice: that members of the board should be 'practising' and not out of touch (Pendry, in HoC, 1992b: 24). David Hinchliffe was one of the two lay appointees on the General Medical Council (Hinchliffe, in HoC, 1992b: 13–14). Hinchliffe had experience of the ENB refusing to validate a training institution because the standard was not high enough. He believed that the ENB had a track record in ensuring that appropriate facilities existed for training and thus did protect the interests of National Health Service patients. He did not want any outside regulation of the boards (Hinchliffe, in HoC, 1992b: 27). In response, Bottomley proposed that National Boards should be national bodies charged with operating the written rules made by the elected body, the UKCC (Bottomley, in HoC, 1992b: 28).

But, as Hinchliffe admitted, he was no expert on nursing: 'I do not pretend to be an expert on nurse training and education, although I am aware of current developments.' He wanted the boards to be independent of government in their monitoring functions. and was concerned that proposed changes by the government would apply merely to educational institutions such as polytechnics, colleges and universities, and not to 'individual hospitals and wards'. He was concerned that the current involvement of the boards with day-to-day experience of nurses training on wards would be removed by the changes in the Bill. This would leave a huge gap between the protection of the interests of nurses in training, which the board would do, and the objective monitoring of the care delivered by the health service. The interests of patients would have no agency to protect them (Hinchliffe, in HoC, 1992b: 29). Hinchliffe seemed to believe that the function of the boards should have some responsibility for objective and independent monitoring of standards of patient care. But the UKCC and the National Boards were, since their inception, entirely independent from hospital administration.

Hinchliffe, it seems, was unclear as to the role of the National Board in relation to nursing schools and hospitals and academic institutions, and the Secretary of State did not answer Hinchliffe's concern. Instead she talked about proper mechanisms in the health service for people to make complaints. The boards were merely to provide 'a point of focus in implementing UKCC rules approving institutions of education'. She did not envisage that they would assume the wider role advocated by Hinchliffe (Bottomley, in HoC, 1992b: 29–30).

Hinchliffe had put his finger on the crucial point. He asked what would happen in future if schools of nursing based in hospitals and their wards were not able to offer sufficiently high standards for placement practice for student nurses. If the boards no longer had jurisdiction over such training schools then there would be a reduction of certain safeguards that applied to the standards of nurse training (Hinchliffe, in HoC, 1992b: 30). Bottomley pointed to the responsibility of the boards towards 'proper arrangements' for ensuring the academic content and practice placements of courses under rules established by the UKCC. She took this as an assurance that proper arrangements would be made as part of the boards' function (Bottomley, in HoC, 1992b: 30). She trusted the profession to regulate its own practical training.

Heal focused on post-registration training (Heal, in HoC, 1992b: 31–32). And Bottomley, too, stressed the importance of post-registration training in developing skills and practices to meet changing needs. She accepted that Project 2000, now well underway, 'is a great success and we are pleased with how it has taken off and has carried the confidence of the profession and the service' (Bottomley, in HoC, 1992b: 38).

Heal, for the opposition, referred to the new training method as placing greater emphasis on the nursing model rather than the medical model: 'Instead of seeing a patient as an appendicectomy on a trolley, as some doctors do, he or she should be seen as Jane Smith or as John Evans. The more personalised approach is important. It involves a partnership between a patient and a nurse.' In support of this approach, Heal raised the issue of the 'Patient's Charter', an initiative from the Prime Minister, which stated that all patients had a right to a 'named nurse', who would be their main or primary nurse caring for them during their stay in hospital. Heal argued that if this role was to be successfully implemented, staff needed development and education and the opportunity to update skills and knowledge (Heal, in HoC, 1992b: 40).

Tom Pendry was less optimistic about the change to nurse education. He quoted an internal memo from a health authority which noted serious financial difficulties in implementing Project 2000. The phasing in of Project 2000, Pendry argued, 'has a detrimental effect on certain members of the nursing profession'. He supported this opinion by a letter from nurses at the sharp end reacting to the internal memo. In this letter from nineteen individuals who had started training at a London hospital in 1989, frustration was expressed not only at the shortage of resources, but also at the amount of theoretical content of the course:

Sadly, we are becoming frustrated and demoralised by the ever increasing erosion of facilities, as well as the amount of theoretical input we are now receiving on our course. Representatives of our group have already raised various issues that reflect our concern and discontent with the Education Manager . . . and the Dean of Nursing . . . These discussions have done

nothing, we feel, to prevent further diminishment of the Nurse Education
facilities or of the consistently high standard teaching we once received.
(Pendryin HoC, 1992b: 43)

The letter continued, numerous administrative changes had reduced the
continuity of the student nurses' training and influenced the standard of
teaching in the classroom and on the wards and departments. Most of the
tutors were now based at the college and were difficult to contact.
Arrangements and decisions were made without any discussion or explanation to students and were supposed to be beneficial: 'although we are
having difficulty in comprehending these benefits'.

The students were constantly reminded that they were accountable for
their actions, but their academic role models were not themselves accountable to the students, and did not address students directly in matters that
affected their training and future careers. When students were expected to
assume 'responsibility for their own learning' a more supportive and
reliable decision-making system should have been in place. 'These issues
may appear trivial to individuals who are not directly concerned with
studying teaching or administrating the "practical skills" RGN course'; but
the students wanted the best training possible. Nursing students at what
Pendry calls 'the sharp end of Project 2000' were very concerned about the
standard of their training (Pendry, in HoC, 1992b: 42–43).

Hinchliffe expressed general unease over how the separate roles of the
UKCC and National Boards would divide when there was an allegation of
misconduct related to a nursing school in a clinical environment
(Hinchliffe, in HoC, 1992b: 44).

Maria Fyfe raised a crucial concern: the balance and integration, under
the new system, of theory and practice. She confessed that she knew
nothing about nursing, midwifery or health visiting, although she knew
something about teaching. What she wanted to know was whether any
consideration had been given to class sizes, and also about implications
for teaching methods and qualifications of teaching staff. She understood
that the teaching of any subject involved endless debate on the balance
between theory and practice, but she asked what safeguards there were to
maintain a reasonable balance. She was also concerned about the transfer-
ability of skills and saw pitfalls in the absence of national monitoring (Fyfe,
in HoC, 1992b: 47).

Bottomley's speech resounded with confident rhetoric. She reiterated
government spending and intentions to deliver excellent education and
training. Concurring with Heal, she talked of patients as partners in health
care and at the forefront of minds when delivering health care. Nurses
needed an adequate training, could not be promised jobs after qualification

and retention rates were very good. She admitted problems, but dismissed their significance. There were bound to be teething difficulties with Project 2000 as in any new form of education. Project 2000, 'with a better balance between the classroom and hands-on work, is important for the future of the nursing profession' (Bottomley, in HoC, 1992b: 49–50).

Opposition MPs might have argued that the intention of Project 2000 was *not* to restore a balance between theory and practice, rather it necessarily upset the balance and introduced a dualism by moving nursing training *away from practice* into colleges, and by making students supernumerary. Moreover, her statement that this was for the future of the nursing profession sat awkwardly with the statement that the patient should be at the forefront of minds. As to Fyfe's question and concern, Bottomley thought this highlighted the importance of a multidisciplinary approach to health matters but asserted that the UKCC was responsible for setting general guidelines while National Boards were responsible for their detailed interpretation. National Boards were responsible for monitoring colleges. Health authorities that sent students on courses would need to monitor the practical performance of those students. If a particular college had a major failure rate, health authorities would not want to send students there. Bottomley's supporting evidence on the positive effects of change was exclusively from the nursing bureaucracy: nursing audit, the nursing development unit and other nurse-led initiatives (Bottomley, in HoC, 1992b: 52).

Fyfe was unconvinced by this reply. Young adults who set off on courses for professional training might find that the institution did not set proper teaching standards. This happened in the world of further education where there were wide variations in the standards achieved in colleges and within departments at colleges. She expressed her concerns:

> I hoped that something more positive would be done about failures to achieve a proper professional standard of teaching. It is not enough to say, "We won't bother to send anyone there". People should have the opportunity to train locally, and proper standards of teaching should be enforced.
>
> (Fyfe, in HoC, 1992b: 52–53)

Bottomley merely reiterated that the National Boards would be responsible for 'invalidating institutions' (sic) and scrutinizing their work. They would ensure high standards of training (Bottomley in HoC, 1992b: 53). But the roles of the UKCC and National Boards remained unclear (Hinchliffe, in HoC, 1992b: 53). And Roger Sims was concerned about the mechanisms that the UKCC would implement regarding trained nurses who were considered to fall below reasonable standards (Sims, in HoC,

1992b: 53–54). Bottomley believed that such questions of incompetence would be dealt with under post-registration matters, in debates on PREP (Bottomley, in HoC, 1992b: 54).

An amendment to the Bill, which would be unsuccessful, was moved by Sylvia Heal which would enhance the role of the National Boards as validators of training courses and institutions and monitors of nurse education. Heal noted the Minister's earlier agreement to monitor pre- and post-registration training (Heal, in HoC, 1992c: 387–88). But Bottomley was clear that she did not want the National Boards to be the agency involved in monitoring post-registration training. The NHS had to do its own workforce planning and ensure that training provision was adequate for needs. The role of the boards was different: their job was to accredit institutions and validate courses, to ensure that the standards of professional education of the UKCC were met and to collaborate with the UKCC in the provision of improved training methods. The responsibility for nurses, midwives and health visitors to maintain and develop their professional skills at post-registration level was currently being considered by the UKCC. Pre- and post-registration budgets were being closely monitored (Bottomley, in HoC, 1992c: 388–89).

Sylvia Heal, from the opposition, supported Mrs Bottomley. Project 2000 was an important development that provided a modern nursing profession prepared to meet the new challenges of future medicine and patient care. It resulted in students adopting different learning methods. It implemented a broader-based curriculum encompassing areas previously given less emphasis – such as ethics, philosophy, sociology, psychology and environment. Students also undertook much more academically based work including increased use of library facilities. Heal ignored the issue that had worried Fyfe, her fellow Labour MP – the balance between theory and practice, and indeed the content of the courses in preparing nurses to be competent. Instead, Heal was concerned about the limitation of resources such as library facilities (Heal, in HoC, 1992c: 390).

Bottomley realized the importance for nurses to learn by hands-on experience, but did not realize, apparently, that this new system made hands-on experience marginal. She relied on the boards to satisfy themselves not only about library facilities, but also that there were adequate clinical placements and that the teaching was of a proper standard (Bottomley, in HoC, 1992c: 392).

The debate had involved a consideration of the role and functions of the Central Council and National Boards in the UK, and in particular on the professions' expectation of them. The government would spend £880 million in that year, and the Secretary of State said that the government recognized its duty to ensure overall mechanisms were in place to guarantee an adequate supply of properly trained nurses, midwives and health visitors to meet the health care needs of the nation in the present and future. The statutory bodies needed to be efficient and effective and directly accountable to the professions.

Surprisingly, the need to be responsible for the protection of patients and the public was not expressed as a prime concern by government. Bottomley stated that the series of important measures instigated by her government had recognized and improved the status of nursing. The government had not only listened to and consulted with the three professions but had acted, in so far as possible, in accordance with their wishes (Bottomley, in HoC, 1992c: 393–96). The concern from grass-roots nursing students about their need for a higher standard and more practical training expressed in the letter to Tom Pendry, and the issues about education standards raised by Maria Fyfe, were not followed up in debates. These serious shortcomings would become a central focus in the years ahead.

Further developments 1997–1999

A review and strategy for nursing, midwifery and health visiting

Confidence in the new system was soon put into question. Five years later, in 1997, Mrs Bottomley's successor, Stephen Dorrell, announced the government decision to commission an independent and fundamental review of the current operations of the five statutory bodies created by the Nurses, Midwives and Health Visitors Act 1979: 'This will be a comprehensive study of all aspects of their work, including those issues around determining fitness to practise which go to the heart of the Council's role in protecting the public' (Dorrell, in HoC, 1997: 345). This was eventually undertaken by a consultancy firm from Bristol, JM Consulting. During the two-year period of this review, which reported in February 1999, developments in, and concerns about, nursing continued to be expressed in Parliament and in parliamentary publications.

Within weeks the new Labour government had taken over responsibility for nursing, and was devising a strategy for nursing, midwifery and health visiting. The Secretary of State for Health, Frank Dobson, published a consultation document, *A Consultation on a Strategy for Nursing, Midwifery and Health Visiting*, a Health Service Circular, (NHSE, 1998a) on 20 April 1998. It was signed by the Chief Nursing Officer, Yvonne Moores.

The document proposed a role for the nurse as a public health worker and health promoter. Quoting from the White Paper, *The New NHS: Modern, Dependable* (Her Majesty's Government, CM 3807, 1997: 46), the document stated that the government was keen that the nurse of the future would have an extended role in acute and community services, take on leadership and monitoring roles, be an educator, a manager and a developer of nurse-led clinics, working across organizational and professional boundaries. The government was committed to encourage and support nursing developing in these new extended ways. Yet careful consideration needed to be given as to how the White Paper objectives could be supported:

> not least because concern has been expressed that role development could result in the fundamental aspects of nursing, midwifery or health visiting practice being overlooked and undervalued. The public hold nurses, midwives and health visitors in high regard not only because of their professional expertise and their ability to enable individuals, families and communities to achieve and maintain optimal physical, psychological and social well being, but also because of the quality of their caring. The best care is valued by the public because it is sensitive and responsive, adjusted to meet changes in dependency, circumstances and need. A key **challenge is to ensure that the development of nursing, midwifery and health visiting roles commands public support and values the essential aspects of caring** which are the very foundations of professional practice.
>
> (NHSE, 1998a: 14, para. 3.15)

The document admitted that the public valued the caring role, and it appears to be saying that the public should be encouraged to believe that this role was being supported.

Questions from the Lords on nursing shortages and nursing care

By June 1998, contrary to the earlier confidence of Mrs Bottomley, it was being acknowledged that there were now serious shortages of nurses. Questions were raised in the House of Lords. Lord Morris asked the government 'what action they propose to take to deal with the problems arising from the recruitment, retention and retirement of nurses in the National Health Service' (Morris, in HoL, 1998a: 1539–42). The facts, said Morris, were not in dispute:

> We are facing the worst nursing shortage crisis in 25 years: the first ever shortfall in applications for nurse education places in England. In 1993/4 there were 18,100 applications for 12,000 places. In 1996/7 there were 15,400 applications for 16,100 places. Turnover among registered nurses was 21 per cent in 1997 up from 12 per cent in 1992. Vacancies remain unfilled. One report in 1997 suggested that there was a shortage of more than 8,000 full-time posts across Britain. The Royal College of Nursing

reports that the number of nurses aged over 55 will double over the next five years, with 25 per cent of registered nurses in the NHS eligible for retirement by the year 2000.

(Morris in HoL, 1998a: 1539)

Morris admitted that this sounded like a boring recital, which some might think a needless worry, because nursing was a vocation: 'It will be all right; someone will do something. The government will find some money. After all, nursing is a vocation, is it not?' Nurses would not take industrial action because they cared too much about patients, Morris supposed. But he realized that this was not good enough. It would not do: 'Try being one of those patients and see how you feel.' Morris's own experience of nursing was of nurses 'hurtling about', moving beds, answering telephones, dishing out meals 'like waitresses', making beds, dispensing drugs, or sitting at the nursing station writing: 'endlessly rushing round or writing' (Morris, in HoL, 1998a: 1539).

Lord Morris asked the government for an up-to-date progress report on the £2.25 million initiative by the government on a nationwide campaign to recruit nurses. He realized that to qualify to become a nurse the young person of 18 must undergo a three-year course, given or validated by a university. Although there might be a bursary of £4,000–5,000, earnings on qualification were £12,000, lower than those of his or her contemporaries: 'Those contemporaries,' said Morris perceptively, 'will rarely be called upon to empty bedpans, clean up the incontinent, or mop up vomit in the earliest years of their employment; nor will they often carry life or death responsibility for their clients' (Morris, in HoL, 1998a: 1540).

Higher salary and career development would help, thought Morris. It should not be the case that to gain promotion it was necessary to leave the bedside and move into management or academic work. He proposed a new grade of 'top rank nurse'. But he also recognized that: 'Something must be done about the high drop-out rate in pre-registration training. Some areas report 30 per cent and more' (Morris, in HoL, 1998a: 1540). He referred to the report, *Project 2000: Fitness for Purpose* (examined in Chapter 3), which had considered attrition, and asked the government to be brought up to date on the prospects of the report's recommendations.

For Morris: 'One thing comes through again and again about pre-registration training: practical clinical skills are not sufficiently achieved by the student.' The clinical teacher had gone and senior clinicians had to 'waste their time' teaching new nurses how to do things on the wards. He wondered about an internship for new diplomates at the end of their course. And he knew that new nurses were considered to be autonomous, accountable practitioners from day one.

Morris conjectured whether the possibility discussed in the Project 2000 report, of an entirely new structure for training health service professionals, in which medical students, nursing students, and others, trained together, would remedy the perceived weaknesses: 'those basic elementary things they all need to know, for example how to give injections correctly, and even how to wash hands correctly' (Morris, in HoL, 1998a: 1540–41). Morris had seen 'several dry thumbs' (meaning unwashed hands) in the period he had spent in hospital. An integrated course would raise status and aid recruitment, he thought, implying perhaps a return to some form of apprenticeship system.

Finally, Morris considered the high turnover rate, family-friendly employment policies, and good-will unpaid overtime worked. He was sure that retention of nurses was improved by government initiatives, skillmix, the NHS Direct scheme, nurse-prescribing, primary care groups and clinical governance. He wondered if the retirement problem could be eased by giving nurses in their last decade at work a lighter workload and increased administrative, advisory and mentoring responsibilities: 'I suspect that what most of them want is not power or riches but job satisfaction' (Morris, in HoL, 1998a: 1541).

It seems that Lord Morris had experienced problems during his stay in hospital, and was casting around for the causes. He brought together the issue of the recruitment crisis, and problems in nurse education. Like the Select Committee which had examined the complaints brought by the Ombudsman, Lord Morris expressed a strong feeling that something was wrong, and he sought reasons in the nationwide shortage of nurses and the evidence of problems in lack of clinical skills.

Baroness Cumberlege declared her interest as vice-president of the RCN. Reiterating the view that she had held to in earlier debates, she suggested that nursing was 'as much an art as a science' and proceeded to restate what she called the 'scientific' base of the nurse. By this she meant not 'hard science' but 'good communication, advocacy, supporting carers and understanding complex family relationships as mending broken minds and broken bones'. GPs were recognizing nurses as becoming expert in asthma and diabetic care. She added that with an increasingly elderly population 'we need nurses now more than ever before' (Cumberlege, in HoL, 1998a: 1541–42).

Cumberlege, a Minister in the previous government, who had been instrumental in bringing changing roles to nursing, including nurse-prescribing, proceeded to ask three questions of the government Minister. First, she asked the government how it would fulfil its intention of recruiting more nurses, given that there was a shortfall of applicants to training places and problems in recruitment. Her second question concerned the status of nursing. Given so many more professions for young women to aspire to, competition to recruit to nursing had never been harder. In order to recruit the brightest men and women, an all-degree profession was crucial. Did the Minister agree? Her third question concerned equal opportunity for funded postgraduate education with the medical profession.

Baroness Masham, with real concern, thought that the subject should not be merely a 'dinner hour debate' but should be given the highest priority. She asked the government to treat it with utmost urgency (Masham, in HoL, 1998a: 1542–43). She, too, had experience of nursing. Years previously, when she had broken her back, her life was saved by the skill of doctors and nurses. The matron had been highly respected, and the sisters, who worked on the wards with junior doctors and nurses, knew how to make the patient comfortable. 'Those days have gone' (Masham in HoL, 1998a: 1543). Recently her husband was in hospital for three months. She saw the sister only once, and that was when her husband had emboli in his lungs.

In her experience, senior staff had been removed from the wards and their years of experience lost to the health service. According to the RCN, to gain promotion nurses had to leave the bedside and move into management or academic work. Junior nurses were not given security, or the benefit of experienced senior specialized nurses as a back-up. Nurses could not cope and were leaving the profession. Particularly at night, young, inexperienced nurses had to cope with very ill, sometimes post-operative patients. They were overwhelmed and patients were insecure. Both patients and nurses needed emotional support.

Staff shortages meant that the wrong people could be appointed. Nurses had so many technical pieces of equipment to learn how to use, and temporary staff were not necessarily familiar with them. Could trained technicians be appointed, Baroness Masham wondered, to ease the burden on nurses' time and physical strain? Baroness Masham wondered how recruitment could be improved.

Lord Hunt also noted the dramatic changes in the nursing role in the past few years. He was optimistic that nurses had taken over many of the duties previously done by junior doctors, which was effective, and 'many patients very much enjoy that and support it' (Hunt, in HoL, 1998a: 1544). He believed that the shift towards primary care would enhance the role of nurses and increase the number of practice nurses and nurse practitioners. He wanted primary care groups to give nurses a leading role. These initiatives, he believed, would be the primary aid for recruitment, although family-friendly policies and initiatives to attract nurses back into the profession would help. He admitted encouragement should be given to nurses who wanted to stay at the bedside, but he was advocating leadership and management positions: 'We need more nurses at the top table' leading debate, and defining the future strategy of the NHS.

Baroness McFarlane chose to focus on educational issues as they affected recruitment, retention and retirement of nurses. She noted that since the Lancet Report in 1932 there had been successive reports on nursing at five or ten-yearly intervals. She wondered if it was now time to focus on 'what is happening in the service, in particular nursing education' (McFarlane, in HoL, 1998a: 1545). The report that changed the face of nursing education, she argued, was Project 2000 published in 1986. Since 1989 nurses had been educated in higher education at diploma and degree level. 'Yet I hear criticism of the Project 2000 system and it is timely that we should examine that' (McFarlane, in HoL, 1998a: 1545). The major criticism that McFarlane heard was that the newly registered nurse was no longer a confident practitioner when she came to the ward. The perception was that the amount of clinical practice had been greatly reduced to accommodate academic studies. She had been told by Dame Betty Kershaw that this was a misconception, because 50 per cent of the course was in clinical practice, although often in the community, where the majority of patients were nursed. That was the explanation for nurses being unconfident when they came to the ward. And she, too, wondered about an intern year, recovering the apprenticeship idea.

McFarlane raised two further points. Her second point concerned trust consortia who commissioned nursing education. She pointed out that their main consideration, rightly, was workforce needs and so they strictly controlled the numbers of students. This made it difficult for students to move from the branch of nursing into which they had been recruited into another branch, and presumably might be a disincentive to them continuing on courses. Her third point was that Project 2000 may have created shortages in psychiatric nursing. There was wastage and academic failure in nursing courses generally, and McFarlane believed that this should be addressed. She seemed concerned by the shortcomings now evident in the system she had helped to implement.

Baroness Emerton declared her own interest as chairman of a trust, of the Nurses Welfare Service, and as a nurse on the register of the UKCC: 'Furthermore, I must confess that I was the chairman of the UKCC when Project 2000 was introduced' (Emerton, in HoL, 1998a: 1546). She argued that retention and recruitment were cyclical, but there was 'no doubt that there is a real problem in the NHS'. The government had invested money into more training places, but there was a reduction in the number of entrants. The problem was attracting young and mature people into the nursing profession. Nursing was a caring profession, argued Emerton, and the ethos of caring needed to be developed in young people. Emerton asked the Minister if 'caring skills' could be introduced into the school curriculum: 'I am sure that we all agree that society generally is not a caring society and that we need to influence young people to enter the profession' (Emerton, in HoL, 1998a: 1546).

Baroness Emerton, interestingly, noted the absence of 'caring' in an uncaring society. The question she implied was why, given this absence, people would choose to enter a caring profession. The remedy, she thought, lay in teaching children how to care. But there is a paradox in her request that children should be taught 'caring skills' at school, particularly in the light of the recommendation by a research study on young people's perception of nursing as a career, conducted by Foskett and Hemsley-Brown (1998), which argued that 'caring' be downplayed altogether because children found it an unappealing idea.

Attrition of student nurses was high, students were dropping out of courses, and now that nursing education was in higher education, Emerton suggested, there was a need to examine selection procedures: 'I suggest that research is undertaken into what we are looking for in nurses entering the profession' (Emerton, in HoL, 1998a: 1546). Nurses needed a good academic base, and a good theoretical knowledge too. They needed to correlate that in delivering practical skills. She repeated her belief that a research project was needed into selection techniques. As regards retention, Emerton's final point was to agree that nurses suffered health problems because of stress.

Lord Graham reiterated a similar story to Lord Morris's of his experience as a patient in hospital. 'I think of the frenetic manner in which the servants of the nation, whatever their rank, were looking after their patients' (Graham, in HoL, 1998a: 1547). As a trade unionist he believed in the case for more money for nurses, or at least, an expression of appreciation of the devotion and dedication given by nursing staff. Baroness Amos (HoL, 1998a: 1548–49) declared her interest as non-executive director of University College Hospital, and chair of the Royal College of Nursing Institute. She agreed with the already expressed problems about recruitment and retention, and argued it was a matter of targeting staff and promoting initiatives for flexible, family-friendly policies. She was encouraged by the commitment of nurses. Lord Addington (HoL, 1998a: 1549–50) admitted that he had no experience of hospitals, only of casualty departments, and he was disparaging about doctors. He believed the answer was money. He did not want to see a 'super grade' paid more, but a higher status for all. Having said that, Lord Addington argued that the problem was that of status.

Earl Howe pointed out that initial entries on the UKCC register had decreased by 25 per cent in the last decade. In 1985, student nurses numbered about 71,000, all employed in the NHS. By 1995, there were

40,000 student nurses, not all of them working in the NHS. There were shortages across the board, competition from other professions for potential recruits, and young people saw nursing portrayed unfavourably in the press and elsewhere. Earl Howe supported the widening of nursing skills, which made nursing more attractive and intellectually challenging especially to graduates. In his view, the entry portals to the profession needed widening, and school children needed to be targeted by 'the projection of a positive image of nursing and patient care' (Howe, in HoL, 1998a: 1550–51).

Earl Howe argued that nurse retention was variable in different areas, and believed that family-friendly policies, automatic clinical updates, professional development and career progression all encouraged retention. He called for free re-entry courses to encourage returnees. To alleviate stress on qualified staff, he believed that ways should be examined closely of 'improving the skill level of health care assistants, to enable them to take on greater responsibilities. The best way is a national register of qualified health care workers, to act as a lever for raising standards in hospitals and social care generally' (Howe, in HoL, 1998a: 1551).

Answering for the government, the Minister, Baroness Jay, spoke of the 'huge variety of roles that nurses undertake every day of the year'. However, 'we all recognise that there are problems and tensions. We know that there are very real issues to address' (Jay, in HoL, 1998a: 1552). The consultation on the strategy of the nursing, midwifery and health visiting professions was underway. And she continued to reiterate the government policy initiatives, such as nurse practitioners, and nurses having more responsibility, for example, by being able to develop triage systems. Jay believed that increased career prospects, leadership positions and status would increase nursing retention and recruitment. She also spoke of more money invested in training and new funding arrangements for students. She reported 14,000 responses to the publicity campaign.

Implying the values of public service were absent or lost, Jay argued for new approaches to their inculcation. To inculcate the 'values of public service', there would be a competition in schools with the idea of 'challenging negative and traditional stereotypes about health service employment, raising awareness about NHS career opportunities and encouraging a broad range of applicants from across society' (Jay, in HoL, 1998a: 1553). Jay was also concerned about 100,000 nurses on the UKCC register who were not working, and money was to be spent on return-to-practice initiatives. Trusts were being encouraged to share ideas, and the telephone service, NHS Direct, was a success, and a way of attracting and retaining nurses in a less stressful job.

Finally, Baroness Jay spoke of listening, promoting health, dealing with racism, developing family-friendly policies and encouraging staff to speak out about their concerns regarding professional standards. She also wanted policies that would reduce stress, and initiatives to promote well-run clinical placements, flexible hours, continuing professional development, encouragement and support from managers and less bureaucracy. She commended the skill and dedication of nurses: 'key components in maintaining the trust we want the public to enjoy into the next century' (Jay, in HoL, 1998a: 1556).

Within a few weeks of this debate in the Lords, Baroness Jay was having to answer critical questions from another peer, Lord Stoddart, about whether the Patient's Charter would be rewritten to ensure nurses did not call patients by their first names (Lord Stoddart, in HoL, 1998b: 75; 8 1998c: 143). According to Stoddart not only patients but also an older generation of nurses were expressing concerns at this failure to accord dignity. Stoddart, a Labour peer, had campaigned under the previous government for the ending of mixed-sex wards, and now he was continuing a struggle to preserve traditional values.

According to Lord Stoddart (1998, personal communication), the response he received was 'overwhelmingly in favour of less familiarity in professional relationships, and in particular against the use of Christian names in the NHS unless the patient wishes it and gives express consent'. The issue of first names, raised by Lord Stoddart, was not a side issue but reflected the changes in nursing and the power struggle involved over changing values and attitudes. This coincided with changes to uniform, and even the loss of uniform, to make the nurse appear more informal, as Rivett (1998) has observed.

That the results of 'informal relationships' were now coming before the UKCC as cases of abuse of patients and inappropriate relationships between patients and practitioners is extremely significant (UKCC, 1998c: 9). The education of nurses *de facto* prepared them for relationships that were 'inappropriate': nurses themselves were torn between what they learned from ideological theories of emotional attachment, and what in reality was right for patients themselves, their needs and desires. Concerns about the appropriateness of the nurse–patient relationship were being voiced at the highest level.

Fifty years of the NHS

In July 1998, in a debate in Parliament on the fiftieth anniversary of the NHS, the Secretary of State for Health in the new Labour government, Frank Dobson, told the House of Commons that NHS staff needed education, training and re-training to be technically competent:

We all still expect nurses to provide tender loving care. These days we also
expect them to cope with using highly complex, hi-tech equipment. They
cannot be expected to do that without the necessary training and time for
training, including training specific to new equipment. When we took
office, we discovered that there is no machinery in the NHS to set performance standards or ensure that they are delivered. Without those arrangements, things go wrong. Nothing is done; people die.
(Dobson, in HoC, 1998b: 1254)

Dobson referred to the new monitoring and standard-setting institutions
that he would soon set up under clinical governance (NHSE, 1998b).
The National Institute for Clinical Excellence was intended to provide
authoritative guidelines for all health professionals, and the Commission
for Health Improvement would monitor the performance of every part
of the NHS (Dobson, in HoC, 1998b: 1254). He commended the work of
those in health care over the past 50 years using the language of
vocation:

Today, we salute the people who work in the NHS – people of all colours,
of all races, of all religions and of none. For every minute of every hour of
every day of the past 50 years, they and their predecessors have bound up
the wounded, healed the sick, cared for the afflicted, comforted the dying
and consoled the bereaved . . . They have fought the good fight . . .
(Dobson, in HoC, 1998b: 1255)

He repeated Bevan's founding philosophy, that the NHS had a spiritual
purpose:

Society becomes more wholesome, more serene, and spiritually healthier,
if it knows that its citizens have at the back of their consciousness the
knowledge that not only themselves, but all their fellows, have access,
when ill, to the best that medical skill can provide.
(Dobson, quoting Nye Bevan, in HoC, 1998b: 1255)

The founding values of the NHS were the same vocational values that had
underpinned nursing, and Dobson assumed them to be changeless. As
Dobson affirmed, nurses were still expected, at heart, to provide tender
loving care. Here was a parallel with Bevan's own purported view of
nursing, that a nurse not working at the bedside was not a real nurse
(Hector, 1972).

Virginia Bottomley, once an enthusiastic and confident defender of the
new system and now in Opposition, pointed to serious problems in the
nursing profession:

> Mention has been made of the recruitment of doctors, but the recruitment
> and motivation of nurses is more important still. There are real difficulties
> in the nursing profession, and I urge the Secretary of State to give priority
> to considering how we can make nursing a long-term, rewarding career.
>
> (Bottomley, in HoC, 1998b: 1276)

Indeed, concerns with nursing were now acknowledged openly. This was
apparent from the report of the review on nurse regulation, published on
9 February 1999 (JM Consulting, 1998b) and accepted by the Labour
government (NHSE, 1999a). The Nurses, Midwives and Health Visitors Act,
established in 1979, amended in 1992 and consolidated in 1997 was to be
repealed. The four National Boards and the UKCC were to be disbanded,
because they failed to protect patients or adequately educate nurses
(*Guardian*, 1999b: 5; *Nursing Times*, 1999a: 5). There was to be a new,
single UK-wide statutory body with ultimate responsibility for setting and
monitoring standards of education, and new educational quality assurance work, to be commissioned by the new Council (NHSE, 1999a).
Protection of the public, by ensuring fitness to practise, was to be the key
function of the new body.

The government established a Change Management Group to address
the practical and policy issues arising from the transition of the five-body
structure (the UKCC and four National Boards) to one regulatory body
(UKCC, 1999e). Standards for nurse education were therefore recognized
to be problematic.

The debate on the Health Bill in the House of Lords, 1999

The government proposed new replacement legislation, which opened the
way to change the regulation of the nursing profession. In the House of
Lords, the government's announcement was made by Baroness Hayman,
the Under-Secretary of State at the Department of Health. Hayman made
clear that the existing systems of professional self-regulation needed to be
strengthened, to become more open, responsive and publicly accountable.
New arrangements for the regulation of nursing, midwifery and health
visiting were needed in order to put public protection explicitly at the heart
of regulation (Hayman, in HoL, 1999a: 109–14). This seems to have been an
admission that the nursing profession had moved away from this function of
regulation, once primary, and, indeed, its original intention.

In the debate that followed, both Baroness McFarlane and Baroness
Emerton spoke to commend the advancement of the profession and to
support the system of regulation that was in place, although they both
appreciated that some strengthening was needed (McFarlane and

Emerton, in HoL, 1999a: 142–44, 165–67). They did not, however, refer to the current problems besetting nursing. These problems were detailed by Baroness Berners (HoL, 1999a: 173–75), who was herself 'a lapsed hands-on nurse'. She referred to the understaffing, but argued that it was important to recruit the right sort of candidates, and moreover to remedy the present lack of practical and compassionate care:

> So yes, we need more nurses, but let us be choosy about recruitment. How carefully are prospective students vetted? There have been reports of a few lazy, insubordinate and intimidating staff in hospital wards. I feel that there should not be an indiscriminate choice of candidates to make an impressive statistic. We are lacking a grade of nurses trained by the bedside both clinically and compassionately, bringing out the practice of common sense for the relief of suffering, including a concern for the anxieties of patients suddenly whisked out of their homes and into unfamiliar surroundings.
>
> (Berners, in HoL, 1999a: 174)

Reforming nurse education

A more coherent system was now acknowledged to be necessary. In a statement to Parliament in 1999, the Secretary of State for Health, Frank Dobson, announced that he intended to reform nurse education. Many nurses and managers recognized that its academic nature did not prepare nurses practically and deterred potential recruits. The move into higher education had broken links with hospitals to the detriment of students and hospitals:

> Many nurses, when they qualify, think that they lack the practical skills necessary on a ward. The transfer of responsibility to the education sector from the health service has broken the old links between individual hospitals and nurses in training, to the disadvantage of both. Many nurses and nurse managers recognise the need for change, so I hope to carry the profession with us – but reform there must be.
>
> (Dobson, in HoC, 1999a: 36)

Ann Keen (HoC, 1999a), an MP and a former nurse herself, blamed the previous government for having 'evicted' nurse training from hospital sites and for moving it into higher education. Most surprisingly, Virginia Bottomley herself (HoC, 1999a: 44) thought reform was now necessary. Project 2000 had merit but it discouraged and disappointed others who wanted training 'for what is ultimately a practical task'. Dobson agreed that the disadvantages of Project 2000 now outweighed the advantages (HoC, 1999a: 44–45); and even Bottomley admitted that the academicization of nursing that her government had introduced with Project 2000 was a mistake (Bottomley, 1999).

Meanwhile, the House of Commons Health Committee, which had been set up to investigate NHS staffing requirements, issued its report (HoC, 1999e). It presumed without question that academic preparation was fitting nurses with technical and technological skills, but admitted nursing students needed to experience more clinical placement. Suggestions to deal with the current staffing crisis included nurses taking on more medical work, and being themselves replaced by a new breed of registered 'assistant nurse'. This marked a recognition that nursing roles were changing, and would entail an urgent response from both inside and outside the profession.

In the summer of 1999, in a debate on health care in Parliament initiated by the opposition, the government confirmed its attitude and approach towards nursing: to improve the status, training, pay and job opportunities of Britain's half million nurses, midwives and health visitors (HoC, 1999c: 1032).

The Health Act received Royal Assent on June 30, 1999. This enshrined for the first time the duties not only of care but also of quality, to be monitored by the Commission for Health Improvement (Health Act, Explanatory Notes, 1999: 37–38, Section 18, paras. 172–74). The Act also made provision for the self-regulation of the health care and associated professions, with regard to the regulatory body, the register of members, the education and training prior to admission to the register, privileges of members, standards of conduct and performance, discipline and fitness to practise, investigation by and enforcement of the regulatory body, appeals, and default powers by a person other than the regulatory body. But the Act also stated that this power could be amended or repealed. The Act affirmed the abolition of the UKCC, and accepted a majority of professionals on the new regulating body when it was formed (Health Act, 1999: 89–90, Schedule 3, paras. 1–8).

Although this was under review, the UKCC had no powers to deal with professional incompetence (National Consumer Council, 1999). Its power was to deal with professional misconduct, but this power had not been used effectively. Towards the end of 1999, the House of Commons Health Committee debated the accountability to the public of the health care professions (House of Commons, 1999f, g). Evidence to the committee concerned nursing care (Elder, in House of Commons, 1999g: 116–17), as well as medical care. The Committee concluded from the evidence that the professions relied too much on individual responsibility, and wanted a more corporate culture of organizational responsibility (House of Commons Health Committee, 1999e: xxiii, para. 23). With regard to nursing, the committee called into question the majority nurse representation on the new Nurses' Council, which was to be in place by September 2001, and suggested instead there needed to be majority lay representa-

tion (House of Commons Health Committee, 1999e: xxxiii, paras. 63–65).
Some witnesses, in particular patients and their relatives and carers, felt
the privilege of self-regulation should end: 'They argued that doctors and
nurses were not properly accountable and "looked after their own".'

This perception that not only the medical profession but also now the
nursing profession could not be trusted to put service above self-interest
marked a fundamental change in the public perception of the nursing
profession, and its 'angel image' from two decades earlier. But there had
been forewarnings. Ann Winterton, for example, in 1992 had argued for
the common sense input of lay representation on the nursing council, and
was worried about the tendency for professions to be 'incestuous',
looking after themselves rather than patients (Winterton, in HoC, 1992b:
14). Bottomley had dismissed this at the time.

The role and purpose of the nurse: reaching the year 2000

Confusion at the heart of nursing

There was now a confusion at the heart of nursing. The variety of course
documents provided by higher education institutions for their degree
courses that were validated by the ENB (Robinson and Leamon, 1999),
revealed a profound dysfunction. These documents showed fragmentation and incoherence in nursing courses. The lack of a common core
curriculum or set standard for registered nurse preparation reflected this
confusion: it was not clear what the job of a nurse actually now was.

The government document *Making a Difference*, published in July
1999, symptomized this incoherence and ambivalence. On the one hand it
suggested a career structure for nurses that embraced the role of nurse
consultant, but on the other hand it highlighted the need to 'increase the
level of practical skills within the training programme' and to 'deliver a
nurse training system that is more responsive to the needs of the NHS'
(Department of Health, 1999: 24, para. 4.4). The DoH document also
stated that the NHS needed to know that nurses were trained to broadly
the same standards and would have the same skills – wherever they were
trained. Nationally consistent benchmark standards for nursing and
midwifery needed to be developed and agreed in partnership with statutory bodies, higher education and the Quality Assurance Agency:

> A consistent approach to pre-registration nurse education is also needed if
> we are to open up more flexible pathways into and within nursing careers.
> Threshold standards for entry to the profession are the responsibility of the
> UKCC, but we propose to agree outcomes for the end of each of the three

years of the education programme in England to ensure that there is a greater consistency in the knowledge and skills that students have at the end of each year of the educational programme.

(Department of Health, 1999: 29, para. 4.18)

But what were nurses being prepared to do? In fact, this document affirmed the traditional functions of nursing as core to the nursing role, and admitted that there were currently lapses in this role:

In some cases fundamental and essential aspects of care, including basic hygiene and mouth-care, tissue viability, nutrition, continence, privacy, dignity and the safety of people with mental illness, have been identified as falling below acceptable standards. Yet these are considered to be core elements of the nursing function and are crucial to patient well-being and recovery.

(Department of Health, 1999: 49, para. 7.9)

The government paper, however, seemed unclear about whether nurses were to be trained by apprenticeship or educated in the liberal arts tradition. Both terms, 'training' and 'education', were used in the document to refer to nurse preparation. This ambivalence appears to reflect an increasingly hazy perception of the registered nurse's purpose and function. June Clark, professor of nursing in Wales, argued that acute hospital nursing should not be part of basic nurse preparation but be a post-basic speciality course. Instead, basic preparation should concentrate on community and primary health care (*Nursing Standard*, 1999b: 7). It may be that the government was more concerned to introduce a form of 'managed care', as was prevalent in North America, a care delivery system which involved telemedicine and greater use of non-doctors (Rivett, 1998: 454). Nurses were certainly being used in this way by the government initiatives.

The nursing leadership, having pressed for the new order of nursing, welcomed the proposals. The Royal College of Nursing described the government proposals as a 'breakthrough document'. There were to be better careers and wider roles for nurses, and already 23,500 (sic) nurses were being trained to take on the responsibility of nurse-prescribing (Denham, in HoC, 1999c: 1026–27).

The government response to the UKCC Commission on nurse education, discussed in Chapter 3, came in the form of a circular to nursing NHS leaders, leaders of nursing organizations as well as educational bodies (NHSE, 1999b) in the autumn of 1999. The Commission report was welcomed because it was in line with the government report *Making a Difference*, complementing and building on it. The letter from the Secretary of State, Frank Dobson, included in the circular stated that 'from the time I took on this job I have been concerned to secure practical changes in nurse education', and he had expressed this concern and outlined the government's priorities for change to the chairman of the UKCC Commission, Sir Leonard Peach. These priorities were: more flexible career pathways into and through nursing and midwifery education; an increased emphasis on practice within the nursing programme; and a nurse education system that was more responsive to the needs of the NHS (NHSE, 1999b: 12, Annex A).

The circular proposed pilot sites to put these priorities into effect. Curricular changes were envisaged, to include an outcomes-based approach with a competency framework; a one-year foundation and two-year branch programme; more flexible entry points to pre-registration nurse education; explicit standards, outcomes and supervision to be set for students; a portfolio of practice experience to demonstrate a student's fitness to practise; a review of the existing practice focus of pre-registration nurse education programmes and to introduce where necessary a stronger practice focus; the facilitation of interprofessional learning and practice; proposals for undertaking, monitoring, evaluating and sharing of good practice (NHSE, 1999b: 15–16, Annex C). The circular also proposed the development of vocational training centres, and 'cadet' schemes.

Seemingly, the government still assumed basic personal care should remain part of registered nurse training, because the circular (NHSE, 1999b: 14, Annex B) set out proposed core competencies for assessment of first-year students. These included: helping patients/clients eat and drink, access and use toilet facilities, maintain personal hygiene and appearance, and be comfortable; mobilizing as planned, as well as performing basic cardio-pulmonary resuscitation; contributing to raising awareness of health issues; understanding the ethical and moral dimensions of care. This list of 24 proposed examples of outcomes was intended for discussion. It was not definitive, and some statements were vague: for example, 'Contribute to the assessment, implementation and evaluation of patient care', and 'Understanding of evidence-based practice'. Nevertheless, by this list the government showed its intention to define some core competencies that were outcome based and were realistic and achievable.

The *Nursing Standard* (1999d: 6) and *Nursing Times* (1999g: 5) reported the circular as asking nursing unions, education heads, UKCC and NHS managers for advice on the level of competence students should have attained in their first year. Concerns remained within the government. The new Chief Nursing Officer, Sarah Mullally, in her inaugural lecture, admitted that nursing education needed to be improved, and that nursing students needed support in clinical practice (*Nursing Times*, 1999h: 6). By the new year, senior nurses at the Department of Health were being charged by the government to set 'benchmarks' for clinical practice in basic hygiene and mouth care; tissue viability (including pressure ulcers, leg ulcers and wound care); privacy and dignity; safety of clients with mental health needs; self-care; record keeping; continence; and nutrition (*Nursing Standard*, 2000a: 5). There were no such national standards in existence.

Alan Milburn, the new Secretary of State for Health, reflected the central issues when he stated that he was keen to break down old professional demarcation borders in health care. Yet education and training of nurses should be driven by the needs of the health service rather than the needs of professional roles. He also wanted to increase skills levels in nurses and create an education system fitting the needs of the NHS and of patients, 'not the other way around'. This meant ensuring national standards: 'Patients, just like NHS employers, need to know that a nurse trained in the north of England has acquired the same level of practical skills as one from the south, at the same stages in nurse training'. In fact, the 'new model of nurse education' was due to start in September 2000 at 16 pilot sites.

The sites would 'focus on the development of practical skills, earlier on in training, in better clinical placements, with better support from trained nurses with good teaching skills, and from nurse teachers who practice [sic] nursing'. Milburn wanted more practising nurses to practise and teach, without being lost from the NHS. The NHS was spending £1 billion on nurse education, and Milburn affirmed that the NHS needed more control on education to ensure consistency, and involve the NHS with professional and regulatory bodies. He wanted to implement an education quality assurance system 'with more bite: a streamlined system to assess fitness for purpose, fitness for practice, and fitness for award'. He also proposed streamlined regulation to promote accountability, 'dealing more effectively with misconduct, poor performance and health issues'. The new Nurses' Council would be in place by September 2001 (Milburn, 1999).

According to the *Guardian*, on the one hand Milburn was keen for nurses to take on doctors' work, while on the other he wanted to restore practical vocational skills to the many 'bread and butter' nurses now being lost. Nursing education needed to fit nurses for the needs of the NHS: 'The curriculum has been determined too much by the professional bodies and universities' (*Guardian*, 1999d: 10). The *Nursing Times* (1999i: 5) and *Nursing Standard* (1999g: 5) reported the speech as advocating nurses taking on more of the work currently performed by doctors, health care assistants doing hands-on nursing, and a new education and training unit at the Leeds-based NHS Executive to develop the delivery of nurse education. Indeed, *Nursing Standard* reported a pilot project to regrade nurses and junior doctors as having government backing. That care assistants were increasingly taking over nursing work was already clear, as evidence documented in Chapter 5 has shown.

But Milburn was keen to 'liberate nurses' as he told RCN Congress later the following year. He was persuaded by the leaders of the nursing profession to widen the remit of nurses, and he listed ten new areas of potential responsibility. These included ordering diagnostic tests, making and receiving referrals, admitting and discharging certain patients, managing a caseload, running clinics, prescribing medicines and treatments, carrying out resuscitation procedures, performing minor surgery, triage for patients and leading in the running of local health services (Milburn, 2000).

Yet a UKCC report which reviewed *The Scope of Professional Practice* (UKCC, 2000a) found concern amongst nurses about widening of their role. While the report's writers saw benefits in boundary blurring, they recognized the need to safeguard what was intrinsic to nursing. Nurses themselves were confused about the logic behind extending roles, increased workload and stress, and managers were worried about issues of accountability. This finding was echoed in another study, which found that parameters of practice were unreliably specified, affecting the assessment of practice skill at all levels (Ashworth, Gerrish, Hargreaves, McManus, 1999).

The government continued to push for expanded and extended nursing roles and professional boundary changes (Department of Health, 2000: 22, para. 4.20). The Royal College of Physicians (2000) reinforced the government policy of breaking down barriers, as did a joint edition of *Nursing Times* (Salvage and Smith, 2000a: 24) and the *British Medical Journal* (Salvage and Smith, 2000b: 1019–20). which included an editorial by Celia Davies (2000a). Salvage and Smith also supported Celia Davies's proposition that what must go was the stranglehold of gender thinking, the root of 'old doctor–nurse stereotypes'.

Celia Davies remained influential. Later that year she published a document on the regulation of the health care professions which was commissioned by the Royal College of Nursing (Davies, 2000b). In it she argued that the present system of professional self-regulation was unsatisfactory and fragmented. She proposed a new model to reduce the power of the professions. This proposal seems ironic, given Davies's own part in the professionalization and empowerment of nursing. However, she downplayed her role in the formation of modern nursing in her history of the UKCC, commissioned by the UKCC, and published in 2000 (Davies and Beach, 2000). This irony was noted, however, by the Unison leader, Paul Chapman (2000), in his review of the book. It is clear that the influence of Davies's ideas, central to the introduction of Project 2000, was maintained.

Although not fully admitting it in her book, Davies did express deep concerns in a subsequent article in *Nursing Standard* in which she was described as being 'one of the architects of Project 2000'. In fact, she confessed to being 'rattled':

> As project officer on Project 2000, it was my job to pull the debate together, and then to go out with my nurse and midwife colleagues to explain it to the profession, the press and the politicians. So how does it all look now?
>
> Project 2000 nurses, at the point of registration, have not got the practical skills. The research bears this out, though it also says they are better grounded theoretically and more adaptable than their predecessors. Academia wants one thing, the NHS another – and educational contracting has not helped. But it was when I started to read the policy documents that I was really rattled.
>
> (Davies, 2000c: 24)

The profession that Davies had encountered in 1986, she said, was reeling from the negatives of what she calls 'service capture and the apprenticeship training that went with it'. Students were 'pairs of hands' and newly qualified staff were insecure. But it was not the whole truth to claim that professionalizers paved the way for academic take-over. Rather, she claimed, the form that Project 2000 had taken was not what was intended. The move to higher education was a by-product of another agenda, the creation of trusts: 'Nursing never makes policy in circumstances of its own choosing.' Notwithstanding her albeit unconvincing defensiveness, Davies admitted that nursing now had to turn back towards service requirements.

But did nurses now have the competence to cope with new roles given problems in the past? Perhaps the government would ensure that nurses reached concrete standards of competence. The Unison Professional Officer, Paul Chapman, was pessimistic about the government drive to define 'competencies'. He thought that the profession would take over, redefine them in line with the current approach, and there would be no real change from the present system. Competencies would remain 'broad-brush' and each institution would define its own competencies locally. There would be no national standard or explicit and transparent detail as the Secretary of State had required in his 1999 keynote speech (Chapman, 1999: 14–15).

Chapman was prescient. The UKCC competency list was drafted for the first year of pre-registration nurse education and sent out for comment by the NHS Executive in February, 2000 (NHSE, 2000). They were broad brush and undefined, as Chapman predicted. The Council used the term competence to 'describe the ability to practice [sic] safely and effectively without the need for direct supervision'. With this definition, competence was divided into four domains: professional/ethical practice, care delivery, care management, and personal/professional development. Outcomes and competencies for each domain were general. Little detail was given. For example, the statement under the domain of care delivery required nurses to contribute to 'the development and documentation of nursing assessments by participating in comprehensive nursing assessment of the physical, psychological, social and spiritual needs of patients/clients'. They should also demonstrate 'essential nursing skills to meet individuals' needs, which include: maintaining dignity, privacy and confidentiality; effective observational and communication skills, including listening; safety and health, including moving and handling; essential first aid and emergency procedures; emotional physical and personal care' (NHSE, 2000: Appendix). These were published by the UKCC in May 2000 (UKCC, 2000b).

Competencies remained vague and abstract, so that, for example, blood transfusion standards were not mentioned, even though an annual report (Serious Hazards of Transfusion, 2000: 6), found that for 'the third year running the most important single cause of mis-transfusion was failure of the bedside checking procedure immediately prior to administering the transfusion'. And this was the responsibility of nursing staff. Infection control was not referred to, even though the National Audit Office (2000) found that 9 per cent of inpatients had hospital-acquired infections. There was no mention, either, of meeting patients' need for nutrition, even though this was widely recognized to be problematic.

The problem that 'nursing' was itself not defined had serious consequences. In a House of Commons debate on the standards of long-term care for the elderly, the proposition of the Royal Commission that the elderly should have free nursing care was responded to by the Health Secretary with the statement that 'nursing care' itself needed definition (Milburn, in HoC, 1999h: 452). Responding to reports of inadequate nursing care for elderly patients, the RCN stated in a press release that the 'essentials of patient care – nutrition, hygiene, dignity, and privacy – are still at the heart of nursing' (RCN, 1999b). However, the nursing job was no longer clearly identifiable. The nature of professional nursing was confused. Arguably, this fragmentation in the nursing role was brought on by the professional leadership itself as a consequence of the quest for status. But now it faced even more fundamental change from the government. Not only was nursing identity in flux but self-regulation and the consequent reliance on personal accountability, the heart and impetus of

Project 2000, had also become the subject of doubt. Poor hospital hygiene was symptomatic (HoC, 2000). It might be that external regulatory controls would be the result (*Daily Telegraph*, 1999b: 1).

The fact that the nursing purpose was now so indistinct was further shown by a House of Lords debate in January 2000, that followed up Lord Morris's earlier concerns. Baroness Masham was worried and perplexed by low standards of nursing. A friend, a patient at a London teaching hospital, was sworn at by a nurse: 'What are we teaching the modern day nurse? Have our standards fallen so low?' (Masham, in HoL, 2000a: 1578). Lord Harrison experienced such disorganized care as a patient that nurses were constantly asking what was wrong with him: 'In my case there also appeared to be a lack of understanding about the care of diabetics injecting insulin' (Harrison, in HoL, 2000a: 1572). Lord Morris, who had instigated this debate, was covered in bruises from subcutaneous injections of anti-coagulants badly given by nurses and he wondered about the quality of current nurse teaching (Morris, in HoL, 2000a: 1575–78).

The nursing members of the House of Lords admitted to problems in nursing practice and education. Baroness McFarlane, Baroness Emerton and Lord MacKenzie expressed concerns about the division of theory and practice. Baroness Cox linked nurse training with teleology, the nursing purpose (Cox, in HoL, 2000a: 1564). But what was the purpose? Baroness Emerton affirmed her belief that the role of the nurse remained primarily that of caring for the sick, and she was concerned about the Health Service Commissioner's report that noted shortcomings in 'traditional areas of care' (Emerton, in HoL, 2000a: 1568–71). The government minister who responded in the debate, Lord Hunt, did not refer to the deficiencies, neither was he clear about the nursing purpose when he reiterated the government policy on nursing (Hunt in HoL, 2000a: 1590–95).

A week later, in a debate on the NHS, two speakers, Lord Winston (Winston, in HoL, 2000b: 297) and Viscount Bridgeman (Bridgeman in HoL, 2000b: 300–1) both expressed concerns about Project 2000. Lord Winston thought it well-intentioned but misguided: 'What we need is caring in the hospitals.' Viscount Bridgeman thought it failed to balance the academic and the practical and urged an early government review.

The government's equivocation and confusion about nursing and the nursing role expressed in so many government publications, was also apparent in its national plan for the NHS, *The NHS Plan*, published in July 2000 (Secretary of State for Health, 2000a and b, Cm 4818-I and II). Previously expressed ideas and proposals about changing the nursing role and regulating health care assistants were affirmed in this document. But the plan also recognized that patients were concerned about standards of hospital care. They wanted an authority figure on the wards, whom they called 'Matron'. Moreover, the plan acknowledged the need to ensure nursing competence, by determining, monitoring and maintaining competence.

By August 2000, the ENB reported that the number of nursing students in training had increased by 2,287 (ENB, 2000). The number of entrants to the UKCC register was also expected to increase, but many of these entries were foreign nurses working in the UK from overseas. Meanwhile the number of complaints from patients and relatives to the UKCC was rising. It was confirmed that Project 2000 was to be phased out of all training organisations by the autumn of 2002, and replaced by an updated diploma currently being tested at 10 universities before being rolled out across England (*Nursing Standard*, 2000b: 5; *Nursing Standard*, 2000c: 4; Nursing Standard 2000d: 5; *Nursing Times*, 2000b: 4).

A report on nursing shortages from the King's Fund found that the public perception of nursing seemed to remain relatively sympathetic, although the nursing image was growing more tarnished. Amongst health care staff at all levels, opinions about Project 2000 were polarized. Negative comments suggested nursing had become too academic and theoretical and too classroom based. One chief executive termed Project 2000 'a mistake'. Others thought Project 2000 had been positive in encouraging nurses to be assertive and questioning (Meadows, Levenson and Baeza, 2000: 52-53). 83 per cent of registered nurses questioned in an opinion poll, said that health care assistants were doing nursing work (RCN, 2000a).

While there were more nursing applicants to universities, the number of students who failed to complete their course in the previous year was high at 14 per cent (*Nursing Times*, 2000c: 6). The shortages of nurses persisted. In September 2000, the government admitted, in evidence to the Pay Review Body, that although the number of nurses working in the NHS had increased by 10,000 since 1997, the number of vacancies had risen from 2.8 per cent in March 1999 to 3.7 per cent in March 2000, and that 9,910 posts remained empty (*Nursing Times*, 2000d: 5; *Nursing Standard*, 2000e: 4). Fears continued (RCN, 2000b)

Against this background, in August 2000, the government published a consultation document on its new regulatory proposals. This involved disbanding the UKCC and National Boards and forming a Nursing and Midwifery Council. This document began by referring to the need for ensuring patients were treated by people 'up to the job' (Department of Health, 2000b:1, para.1.1), implying that the need for reform was obvious. Amongst other proposals, the document suggested that the new regulatory body should be responsible for setting the standards of training, admission to training and outcomes to be achieved, and for ensuring that registrants met these standards. Consultations on the future direction of the nursing profession were set to continue over the next year.

In November 2000 the UKCC published its response to the government's proposed changes to regulation. It criticised them as intrusive (UKCC News Online, 2000a). This was despite its own rather defensive admission of a dramatic rise of complaints against nurses, midwives and health visitors (UKCC News Online, 2000b). Meanwhile, statistics showed that the number of unregulated health care assistants had risen by 50 per cent in five years (Incomes Data Services Ltd., 2000). By 1999 there were 25,500 health care assistants (21,400 whole time equivalent posts) in the NHS.

Conclusion

The nursing profession was a focus for political debate in the last decade of the twentieth century. Politicians expressed doubts about whether the new system of nurse self-regulation was protecting the public sufficiently. There was confusion about the role of the UKCC and National Boards. Questions were asked in Parliament about nurse education, whether it was practical enough and how standards were assured. Concerns expressed to politicians by grass-roots nursing students about the deficiencies of their training in practical skills, as well as similar concerns voiced by politicians themselves, were not followed up in debates.

It seems to have been assumed, however, that a model of nurse education of a liberal arts kind was superior to an apprenticeship model. Key to the changes in nursing, as politicians realized, was the status of the profession. Public protection was not central. And politicians trusted the profession and admitted their own ignorance. But the changes in nursing reflected the spirit of the age, marked by feminism and freedom, with associated values of autonomy, flexibility and spontaneity, in reaction to what was perceived as male-dominated hierarchy, regulation and structure.

Concerns were sufficiently strong for the Conservative government to set in train a review of the Nurses, Midwives and Health Visitors Act, specifically to examine the issue of regulation and public protection. While this review was being undertaken, questions were raised in the House of Lords about shortages of nurses and wastage from nursing courses. Members of the Lords who had themselves experienced inadequate standards of nursing care were casting round for the reasons for failures. By 1999, there was recognition by the highest levels of government that nursing was not practical enough and an admission that the nursing profession needed some mechanism of external control.

But there were also contradictions. Politicians were unclear about what they expected the nursing role to be. Some assumed that personal caring was still the key nursing responsibility, while others saw nursing developing into extended roles instead. Pressures from the nursing leadership to increase the status of the nurse seemed to resonate with government policy in managing the NHS and bringing in nurses to address patient concerns, focused by initiatives such as the NHS Direct nursing telephone service. The concern about professional self-regulation, particularly with regard to doctors and what was perceived to be their innate conservatism, may also have affected the increased and expanding nursing role.

Governments seemed ignorant and ambivalent. Nurses were ideal change agents, it was argued, keen on progress, and indeed many were persuaded of the advantages and benefits of this new approach. On the other hand, the government was concerned to reintroduce vocational nursing skills. Paradoxically by the end of the century, traditional caring values seemed increasingly marginal as nurses moved into these new roles and functions, and health care assistants took over traditional nursing work. Yet, simultaneously, nursing accountability and self-regulation were now recognized to be problematic. The principle of individual professional responsibility, introduced at the beginning of the 1980s, had not proved adequate. Moreover, the future of nursing was unclear and its purpose undefined. By the end of 2000, even the health economist Alan Maynard (2000) was to admit that nursing was suffering from serious self-inflicted problems.

CONCLUSION

The paradox of nursing at the year 2000

The chapters of this book have presented evidence from reports, studies, statistics and debates on nursing in Britain since 1978 with the intention to allow the evidence to speak for itself. It is now time to sum up the evidence for the reader, and draw out some of the key implications for the nursing profession and for patient care.

The Nurses, Midwives and Health Visitors Act 1979, introduced in Parliament in 1978, not only set in motion a new structure for the nursing profession in Britain but also ushered in an entirely new ethos. Project 2000 was the characterizing component of this change and defined it. Welcomed, with some provisos, by the Conservative government in 1988, and implemented in 1989, Project 2000 can be seen to have coincided with the spirit of the age. The values of autonomy, creativity, enterprise and spontaneity were pre-eminent in this period in Britain. The mood was against hierarchy, rigid structure and external regulation. There is no doubt that educational theory played a major part in restructuring nursing and nurse education. At the same time, the more managerial and market-driven focus of the NHS meant that it was convenient to sever the links between nurse training and service needs. Change suited both the professional leadership of nursing and the culture of the National Health Service.

Although the plans and proposals of the professional leadership chimed with this culture, they were not welcomed by many grass-roots nurses, for whom the vocational tradition was still very relevant. Nevertheless, disagreement was ignored and the apprenticeship training was replaced by a new educational system, designed to increase the status of nursing as an independent self-regulated profession. Nurses were to be prepared to be autonomous and independent practitioners. The rise of the feminist movement may be relevant background. Vocational values and traditional methods and structures were discounted, dismantled and superseded. Nursing was to move from the vocational to the contractual, paralleling the secularization of society and the displacement of concepts such as vocation. The effects of this change were fourfold.

First, nurse training, and its basis in biomedical knowledge, practical skill and procedure, was replaced by a model of education which focused predominantly on the acquisition of psychosocial techniques. This altered the notion of competence and its achievement. It also shifted the context of learning from the clinical setting and patient care to the classroom and the student learning experience. The prescriptive national syllabus, with its detailed list of learning requirements, including anatomy and physiology, the nature and nursing care of diseases, dietetics and so on, was ended, as was the national state examination of both theory and practice. Also ended was the practical record which accompanied student nurses throughout their training and which listed the practical procedures that demonstrated the nurse's proficiency.

The apprenticeship method of learning to be a nurse was rooted in the context of ward practice. The nurse developed her skills and abilities progressively, through experience on the wards combined with formal classroom lectures and examinations within the hospital. This practice-based training was replaced by a college-based system supplemented with placements. The apprentice nurse became a supernumerary nurse, whose main learning took place away from the hospital ward. The discipline of structured duty was no longer key to her preparation. Individual higher education institutions prepared their own syllabuses and methods for assessment of nursing competence. In consequence, the new educational system brought a dichotomy between theoretical knowledge and practical skill. It also introduced fragmentation and a lack of clarity as to what constituted nursing competence, how it was attained, and how it was tested, at both basic and advanced levels.

Second, the role of the ward sister lost authority and significance. Traditionally the ward sister had been the pivot on which the ward functioned. She had supervised and taught the student nurses, and was responsible for the quality of patient care. Under the new system, nursing students were assigned to individual trained nurses when they came to the wards in a supernumerary capacity. The ward learning experience was unstructured in comparison to the previous system. Formal procedures for performing a bedbath, or performing mouth care, or laying up a dressing trolley and performing a dressing, for example, which had been the responsibility of the ward sister and which followed a prescribed and systematic pattern, were no longer applicable.

Ward routines, instigated and monitored by the ward sister, liberated the nurse from having to think about how to perform basic procedures.

Confident that she or he was competent, the nurse was freed (theoretically, at least) to focus on individual patient needs and personal requirements. The nurse did not then have to worry that he or she might be doing the wrong thing. Ward routines were now discarded in favour of flexibility. The individual qualified nurse became personally responsible and accountable for his or her own practice, and no longer answerable to the ward sister. The ward sister lost the power of supervision that had previously been vested in her by virtue of the authority of her role, and power transferred instead to individual registered nurses with a consequent fragmentation of leadership and standards. Most important of all, the ward sister had been responsible for inducting student nurses into the ethos and associated values of nursing care. The new system had no such internal mechanism, and no longer recognized the same values.

Third, the new system of nursing, with its reconstructed values, had an impact on relationships between colleagues in the medical, nursing and allied professions. The co-operative model of working, which had characterized the traditional system and which was built on a common purpose of service to the patient, was replaced by the individualism and competitiveness of a more market-oriented philosophy. Values of loyalty, trust and mutuality, the professional etiquette which nurses had previously learned in their apprenticeship training, were replaced by values that appealed to autonomy, independence and self-confidence. Obligation and commitment were not owed to medical staff.

The relationship of dependence and subordination between nursing and medicine in what was perceived to be the patient's best interests was no longer considered appropriate. The feminist critique of hierarchical, male-dominated structures, related to criticisms of the medical profession. The nurse could no longer place trust in and devolve responsibility to the doctor. The nurse alone now had responsibility for her actions, both commissions and omissions. For the nursing profession this has involved a movement into new and independent nursing roles that not only make nursing self-reliant, unconstrained by medicine, but also encroach on what was previously the work of doctors. Arguably, this has brought some measure of conflict to the professional relationship, and a liability to increase the anxiety and stress on the nurse, who has no clear way to measure her own level of competence. Market-based pragmatism in the growth of new nursing roles and responsibilities has resulted in their haphazard development, without robust measures for ensuring competence. It has also taken nurses away from what was still for many their *raison d'être* – practical, bedside caring.

Finally, and fundamentally, the reliance on the nurse's moral character, 'a good nurse being a good woman', was no longer seen as relevant to nurse preparation. Contract had replaced covenant as the underlying value system of the nursing profession. Secularism meant that the idea that nursing was a vocation with its quasi-religious significance was unacceptable under the new model of nursing. Even so, many nurses, who were mainly still female, continued to hold this to be their own primary motivation. What had previously defined the nursing role as that of a moral relationship, embracing qualities of self-sacrifice and dedication in putting the needs of patients first, and which had given nurses their value in the minds and hearts of the public, was now deemed at best irrelevant by the profession. The quasi-sacred bond of nurse to patient, grounded in reverence for the sick and suffering person, was commuted into the more functional contractual notion of professional service to the client.

Arguably, the contractual model has been unable to sustain the ethic of compassionate care. The move from covenant to contract had the effect of altering both attitudes and values relating to the tasks performed by the nurse for the patient. The bedpan was no longer the symbol of glory but the symbol of humiliation and servitude. Washing, cleaning away vomit and excreta, or feeding, were no longer seen as acts of virtue crucial to care requiring goodness of character, but menial commodities of relatively low marketable value. The vocational tradition had regarded the body as a temple of the spirit. There was, therefore, no hierarchy between body and soul, and no distinction in value between what might be termed to be personal care and more complex technical or emotional care.

Moreover, by participating in personal care, the nurse could not only observe the patient's physical and emotional condition as a basis for treatment, but was enabled to enter into a moral covenant relationship with the patient, in the most genuine and meaningful way. Without this moral foundation, the new system held there to be a hierarchy of status in the tasks performed and the knowledge and skill needed. This had the effect of making basic nursing care less economically valuable, transferable to less trained workers. Washing the floor, washing a patient, giving out food, or feeding a patient, became tasks which differed little in marketable value. This division of labour has had a profound and continuing effect on the nature of nursing and the quality of what was once deemed to be 'total patient care'.

Five paradoxes, arising from these profound changes, confronted the nursing profession at the start of the year 2000. The first paradox is that of recruitment and retention. The number of registered nurses on the UKCC register fell from 1986, the date of the Project 2000 proposals, onwards. In 1986/87 there were 37,668 admissions to the UKCC register which included 2,577 EC/non-EC admissions. In 1998/99 there were 26,934 admissions to the UK register which included 5,033 EC/non-EC admissions. At the start of 2000, the number of nurses on the register was at its lowest for seven years, with more nurses leaving than joining. Students were dropping out of educational courses, and registered nurses were leaving the profession. Eighty per cent of NHS trusts reported difficulties in recruiting nurses. Notwithstanding that in 1986 recruitment and retention statistics did not warrant changing the system, Project 2000 was confidently expected to improve recruitment and retention and to reduce student wastage in the longer term. The paradox lies in the fact that recruitment and retention of nurses and nursing students has not improved as was intended. Add to this the irony that the new educational system was envisaged as providing nurses with transferable skills that would qualify them for jobs other than nursing.

The second paradox concerns the evidence for radical educational change. The changes to nursing education through the introduction of a predominantly liberal arts curriculum have attracted much criticism, but have been strongly defended by the nursing leadership. What was supposed to be a balance of theory and practice has fulfilled neither aspect satisfactorily, so that nurses were now recognized to be deficient in practical nursing skills at registration. The suggestion of an internship year following registration seemed to be an admission that some mode of apprenticeship learning is necessary to nurture practical caring skills. Some major component of apprenticeship training proves inevitable. It seemed that a 'new model' of nurse education with competencies defined and taught to recognized standards might gradually displace Project 2000 in the new century, although this was far from clear. The paradox is the enthusiastic implementation of fundamental root and branch change to traditional nurse training when there was minimal evidence to justify it – in contrast to the dogged resistance to any major change to the Project 2000 system when the evidence of serious shortcomings for patient care had become overwhelming.

The third paradox is that of regulation. Under the previous system the nursing profession was regulated by statute, and supervised by the ward sister and matron, who assured its quality. The move to total self-regulation by the profession from 1979 onwards, so important to the leaders of the profession for a mixture of motives, has proved brittle. The UKCC and four National Boards were to be disbanded and replaced with a new nursing council. External lay membership of the nursing body was being urged as necessary for the profession to be fully accountable. And the regulatory body of the nursing profession had to be reminded that its primary purpose is public protection. External inspection of NHS wards and departments by a body independent of the profession was deemed necessary. The paradox is that the profession's own internal mechanisms could no longer be trusted, and nursing had now to submit to imposed and external inspection in order to safeguard patient care.

The fourth paradox is that of professionalization and vocation. In order to attract nurses into the profession, recruitment has highlighted 'higher status' work rather than practical basic nursing care. But evidence showed that the vocational imperative of altruism, expressed in personal bedside caring, was the key motivating factor in recruitment and retention. The college-based process of forming a nurse, however, ignored this evidence and discouraged this motivation, replacing it with a drive that was more status-conscious and self-assertive. Unless an ideal is nurtured it weakens. As nursing has become professionalized, and caring has become commodified, the vocational ideal has withered. This paradox suggests that, in a pluralistic age, a variety of paths into nursing and nurse preparation might allow the vocational imperative to remain as at least one path for nurses to choose.

There is another aspect to this paradox, that of public esteem and status. Under the vocational model of nursing the nurse did not aim for status, but in the public mind she was accorded the highest possible esteem because of her altruism. Status rested in the value accorded her as a bedside carer. The new order deliberately broke with this altruistic 'angel image' and sought a higher 'professionalized' status in other roles. As the bedside nurse became less valued by the profession, so the nurse at the bedside of sick and vulnerable people has less public esteem, as the weight of evidence from this book shows. This leads to the fifth paradox.

The fifth paradox is the most important and profound: the purpose of nursing with regard to the centrality of patient care. Quality and consistency of the personal care of older people, particularly for the most frail and vulnerable, who formed the majority of hospital patients, had become a focus of serious criticisms. Arguably, these shortcomings have arisen because the central needs of the patient, once the primary purpose of the nursing profession, have become secondary to the focus on the development both of the individual nurse and the nursing profession that is the mark of 'professionalization'. The profession's had come to define the nature of patient need, rather than as previously when the needs of patients defined the nature of the profession. Further, as the nursing role changed to meet the requirements of status and professionalization, so boundaries between the medical and nursing professions blurred and are likely to continue so. It was now probable that personal care for the patient was performed by health care assistants rather than qualified nurses. The paradox is that health care assistants became nurses in all but name, while nurses were not nursing.

These five paradoxes, the result of remaking British general nursing for the year 2000, have focused vital questions about the value system and ethos which has inspired this radical reconstruction. Whether nursing has the capacity to learn lessons from the experience of Project 2000 remains the key question for the future of patient care and the nursing profession.

References

In keeping with the use of abbreviations in citations in the text, the following abbreviations are used in the references:

ENB – English National Board for Nursing, Midwifery and Health Visiting
GNC – General Nursing Council for England and Wales
HoC – House of Commons
HoL – House of Lords
NHSE – National Health Service Executive
RCN – Royal College of Nursing
UKCC – United Kingdom Central Council for Nursing, Midwifery and Health Visiting

Abel-Smith B (1960) A History of the Nursing Profession. London: Heinemann.
Age Concern (1999) Turning Your Back on Us: Older People and the NHS. London: Age Concern.
Aiken LH, Smith HL, Lake ET (1994) Lower medicare mortality among a set of hospitals known for good nursing care. Medical Care 32(8): 771–87.
Alderman C (1997) Here's looking at you. Nursing Standard 11(16): 23–27.
Allen C (1990) P2000 problems. Nursing Standard 5(6): 43–44.
Allen C (1993) Empowerment, taking chances, making changes. In Dolan B, (Ed) Project 2000: Reflection and Celebration. London: Scutari Press. pp. 57–74.
Allman DJ (1998) NHS needs a degree of sense. The Express (Letters to the Editor), 8 August: 37.
Ashdown AM (1917) A Complete System of Nursing. London: JM Dent and Sons Ltd. (2nd edn, 1922; 3rd edn, 1939; 4th edn, 1943)
Ashworth PD, Gerrish K, Hargreaves J, McManus M (1999) 'Levels' of attainment in nursing practice: reality or illusion? Journal of Advanced Nursing 30(1): 159–68.
Association of Community Health Councils (1997) Hungry in Hospital? Health news briefing, 30 Drayton Park, London, N5: ACHC.
Atkinson E (1998) Degrees of care. Daily Mail (Letters), 11 August: 43.

Audit Commission for Local Authorities and the National Health Services for England and Wales (1997) Anaesthesia under Examination. London: Audit Commission.

Audit Commission for Local Authorities and the National Health Services for England and Wales (1998) The Doctor's Bill: Provision of Forensic Medical Services to the Police. London: Audit Commission.

Audit Commission for Local Authorities and the National Health Services for England and Wales (1999) Critical to Success: The Place of Efficient and Effective Critical Care Services within the Acute Hospital. London: Audit Commission.

Baldwin N (1998) Dignity denied. The Guardian (Society), 29 July: 3.

Barrett J (1997) Nurse education, a time for change. British Journal of Nursing (Correspondence) 6(19): 1136.

Bartlett HP, Simonite V, Westcott E, Taylor HR (2000) A comparison of the nursing competence of graduates and diplomates from UK nursing programmes. Journal of Clinical Nursing. 9: 369–81.

Bedford H, Phillips T, Robinson J, Schostak J (1993) Assessing competencies in nursing and midwifery education. London: ENB.

Bendall ERD (1975) So You Passed, Nurse. London: RCN and NCNUK.

Bendall E (1977) The future of British nurse education. Journal of Advanced Nursing 2: 171–81.

Binnie A, Titchen A (1999) Freedom to Practise. Oxford: Butterworth-Heinemann.

Blegen MA, Goode CJ, Reed L (1998) Nurse staffing and patient outcomes. Nursing Research 47(1): 43–50.

Bliss MR (1998a) Technological medicine and the elderly, who cares? Journal of the Royal Society of Medicine 91(March): 152–53.

Bliss MR (1998b) The anguish of families. Paper read at a meeting of the East London Common Purpose Programme, St Barthomolomew's Hospital, 7 April: 1–3.

Bliss MR (1999) They're no angels. The Spectator, 27 November: 17–18.

Bond S, Thomas LH (1992) Measuring patients' satisfaction with nursing care. Journal of Advanced Nursing 17: 52–63.

Booth B (1996) Old-timer's lament. Nursing Times 92(14): 57.

Bottomley V (1999) World at One, BBC Radio 4, 6 January.

Boyle S (1992) Assessing mouth care. Nursing Times 88(15): 44–46.

Bradshaw A (1994) Lighting the Lamp: The Spiritual Dimension of Nursing Care. London: Scutari Press.

Bradshaw A (1995) What are nurses doing to patients? A review of theories of nursing past and present. Journal of Clinical Nursing 4(2): 81–92.

Bradshaw A (1997) Defining competency in nursing (part I), a policy review. Journal of Clinical Nursing 6: 347–54.

Bradshaw A (1998) Defining competency in nursing (part II), an analytical review. Journal of Clinical Nursing 7: 103–11.

Bradshaw A (In press) The Nurse Apprentice, 1860–1977. Aldershot: Ashgate Publishing.

Bree-Williams FJ, Waterman H (1996) An examination of nurses' practices when performing aseptic technique for wound dressings. Journal of Advanced Nursing 23: 48–54.

Briggs A (1979) The essence of Briggs. Nursing Times 75(9): 345.

Briggs A (1983) The commitment of the Briggs Committee In A Time for Commitment: A one-day conference held on Tuesday 15 November, 1983, Chairman: Baroness Cox of Queensbury, p. 2–9, London: ENB.

Bright M (1997a) She was dying for a cuppa. Literally. The Observer, 28 September: 26.

Bright M (1997b) Charity calls for abuse inquiry. The Observer, 26 October: 18.

Brignall J (1997) Hidden agenda behind push to increase nursing's role. Nursing Times (Letters) 93(20): 20.

British Journal of Nursing (1921) The General Nursing Council for England and Wales. British Journal of Nursing, 2 April: 187–89.

BMJ (1982) Changing relations between doctors and nurses, CCHMS critical of RCN's discussion documents. British Medical Journal (supplement) 285: 1130–32.

BMJ (1983) From the JCC: nursing process criticised. British Medical Journal 287: 439–41.

BMJ (1986) From the CCHMS, Concern at "Project 2000". British Medical Journal 293: 1585–86.

Brookes Y, Bristoll C, Young B (1997) Driving nurses away from caring. Nursing Standard (Letters, West Midlands) 12(12): 10.

Brown DF (1998) Nurses' training. The Scotsman (Letters to the Editor), 8 August.

Buchan J (1997) Magnet hospitals. Nursing Standard 12(7): 22–25.

Buchan J (1998) Employment Brief 21/98: Carry on Nursing? London: RCN.

Buchan J, Seccombe I, Smith G (1998) Nurses' Work: An Analysis of the UK Nursing Labour Market. Aldershot: Ashgate.

Bullivant D (1998) A career in nursing: some negative perceptions. Human Resources in the NHS 23: 10.

Butterworth T (1992) Clinical supervision as an emerging idea in nursing. In Butterworth T, Faugier J, (Eds) Clinical Supervision and Mentorship in Nursing. London: Chapman and Hall. pp 3–17.

Caines E (1998) A hole of your own. Nursing Times 94(36): 40–41.

Caines E (1999) How to end the nursing shortage. The Spectator, 6 September: 6, 11.

Carlisle D (1994) A fresh start. Nursing Times 90(45): 16.

Carpenter M (1978) Managerialism and the division of labour in nursing. In Dingwall R, McIntosh J, (Eds) Readings in the Sociology of Nursing. Edinburgh: Churchill Livingstone. pp 87–103

Carr-Hill R, Dixon P, Gibbs I, Griffiths M, Higgins M, McCaughan D, Wright K (1992) Skill Mix and the Effectiveness of Nursing Care. York: Centre of Health Economics, University of York. September.

Carr-Hill R, Dixon P, Gibbs I, Griffiths M, Higgins M, McCaughan D, Rice N, Wright K (1995) The impact of nursing grade on the quality and outcome of nursing care. Health Economics 4: 57–72.

Cartwright A (1964) Human Relations and Hospital Care. London: Routledge and Kegan Paul.

Casey N, Smith R (1997a) Bringing nurses and doctors closer together. British Medical Journal (Editorial) 314: 617–18.

Casey N, Smith R (1997b) Bringing doctors and nurses closer together. Nursing Standard 11(23): 1.

Castledine G (1994) Specialist and advanced nursing and the scope of practice. In Hunt G, Wainwright P, (Eds) Expanding the Role of the Nurse. Oxford: Blackwell Science. pp 101–13.

Chapman P (1998) Degree of scepticism. Nursing Times 94(3): 63.

Chapman P (1999) Learning swerve. Nursing Times 95(48): 14–15.

Chapman P (2000) Interpreting professional self-regulation: A history of the United Kingdom Central Council for Nursing, Midwifery and Health Visiting, (Review). Nursing Times 96(31): 34.

Charnley E (1999) Occupational stress in the newly qualified staff nurse. Nursing Standard 13(29): 33-36.

Christie R (1999) '. . . but not the right theory.' Nursing Times (Letters) 95(42): 21.

Clark J (1997) Reflection: In my opinion. Assignment – ongoing work of health care students 2(2.3/2.4) University of Manchester, School of Nursing, Midwifery and Health Visiting.

Clark J (1998) An educationalist, a consumer group spokesperson and an independent nurse consultant share their hopes for the review. Nursing Standard 12(50): 54.

Clarke K (1983) The political commitment. In A Time for Commitment. A one-day conference held on 15 November 1983, Chairman, Baroness Cox of Queensbury. London: ENB. pp 49–62.

Clarke K (1989) Letter to Dame Audrey Emerton, DBE, Chairman UKCC. London: Department of Health and Social Security.

Clarke M (1971) Practical Nursing.11th edn. London: Baillière Tindall.

Clinton HR (1994) Speech given to American Nurses Association Convention. San Antonio, Texas, 11 June.

Cochrane DA, Conroy M (1996) The Future Healthcare Workforce. Manchester: University of Manchester Health Services Management Unit.

Cochrane DA, Conroy M, Crilly T, Rogers J (1999) The Future Healthcare Workforce, The Second Report. Bournemouth: University of Bournemouth.

Cochrane M (1930) Nursing. London: Geoffrey Bles.

Council of Deans and Heads of UK University Faculties for Nursing, Midwifery and Health Visiting (1998) Breaking the Boundaries. University of Manchester: Council of Deans and Heads.

Cox C (1993) Closing thoughts on hidden agenda – an epilogue. In Jolley M, Brykczyńska G, (Eds) Nursing: Its Hidden Agendas. London: Edward Arnold. pp 159–71.

Cox C, Lewin D, Hewins S, Bowman K (1983) The Clinical Learning Project. London: Nursing Education Research Unit, University of London.

Croft J (1873) Notes of Lectures at St Thomas's Hospital. London: St Thomas's Hospital, Blades East and Blades.

Cullum N, Dickson R, Eastwood A (1996) The prevention and treatment of pressure sores. Nursing Standard 10(26): 32–33.

Cutting KF (1998) Identification of infection in granulating wounds by registered nurses. Journal of Clinical Nursing 7: 539–46.

Daily Telegraph (1999a) NHS and the elderly (Sandra Laville, Celia Hall). The Daily Telegraph, 6 December: 10–11; 7 December: 14–15; December 8: 4. (Harris, M), 9 December: 10, 30; (Letters), 9 December: 31; (Letters), 10 December: 17, 31; (Letters), 11 December: 25.

Daily Telegraph (1999b) Inspection of wards for elderly "to be a priority". The Daily Telegraph, 13 December: 1.

Dannatt A (1893) How to Become a Hospital Nurse. London: The Record Press Ltd.

Darley M (1999) Poor ward preparation. Nursing Times 95(1): 64. January 6.

Davies C (1990) The Collapse of the Conventional Career. A report for the ENB, Project Paper One. London: ENB. September.

Davies C (1995) Gender and the Professional Predicament in Nursing. Buckingham: Open University Press.

Davies C (2000a) Getting health professionals to work together. British Medical Journal 320: 1021–22.

Davies C (2000b) Stakeholder Regulation: A Discussion Document. London: RCN. June.

Davies C (2000c) Plotting a course. Nursing Standard 15(1): 24.

Davies C, Beach A (2000) Interpreting Professional Self-Regulation: A History of the United Kingdom Central Council for Nursing, Midwifery and Health Visiting. London: Routledge.

Davies L (1999) Do as you would be done by. Nursing Times (Letters) 95(44): 19.

Davis F (1975) Professional socialization as subjective experience, the process of doctrinal conversion among student nurses. In Cox C, Mead A, (Eds) A Sociology of Medical Practice. London: Collier-Macmillan. pp 116–31

Davis M (1997) The killing of Sister Plume. Nursing Times 93(35): 35.

Davison G (1997) Give credit to those with track record. Nursing Standard (Letters) 12(12): 10.

Day H, James P (1997) Such common sense lacking in nursing. Nursing Standard (Letters) 12(10): 11.

Dean M (1992) London perspective, nursing's identity crisis. The Lancet 339: 1160–61.

Delamothe T (1988a) Nursing grievances I: Voting with their feet. British Medical Journal 296: 25–28.

Delamothe T (1988b) Nursing grievances II: Pay. British Medical Journal 296: 120–23.

Delamothe T (1988c) Nursing grievances III: Conditions. British Medical Journal 296: 182–85.

Delamothe T (1988d) Nursing grievances IV: Not a profession, not a career. British Medical Journal 296: 271–74.

Delamothe T (1988e) Nursing grievances V: Womens work. British Medical Journal 296: 345–47.

Delamothe T (1988f) Nursing grievances VI: Other places, other solutions. British Medical Journal 296: 406–8.

Delamothe T (1988g) Nurses make the grade. British Medical Journal 296: 1344.

DeMoro RA (1999) Nurses and quality of care (Part II) Market-based remedies fail. Opposing view. Law will ease nurse workloads, patients' minds. USA Today, 18 October: 18A.

Department of Health (1999) Making a Difference. London: Department of Health. July.

Department of Health (2000a) A Health Service of all the Talents: Developing the NHS Workforce. London: Department of Health. April.

Department of Health (2000b) Modernising Regulation - The New Nursing and Midwifery Council: A Consultation Document. London: Department of Health. August.

Department of Health Nursing Division (1998) A Strategy for Nursing: A Report of the Steering Committee. London: Department of Health. April.

Devlin B (1987) An unreal brave new world? Nursing Times 83(18): 29–30.

Dickson N (1987) A top priority. Nursing Times 83(18): 28.

Dingwall R, McIntosh J (1978) Readings in the Sociology of Nursing. Edinburgh: Churchill Livingstone.

Dingwall R, Rafferty AM, Webster C (1988) An Introduction to the Social History of Nursing. London: Routledge.

Domville EJ (1885), A Manual for Hospital Nurses. 5th edn. London: J and A Churchill. (7th edn, 1891; 9th edn, 1907)

Dowling S, Barrett S, West R (1995) With nurse practitioners who needs house officers? British Medical Journal 311: 309–13.

Doyal L, Dowling S, Cameron A (1998) Challenging Practice: An Evaluation of Four Innovatory Nursing Posts in the South-West. Bristol: University of Bristol, The Policy Press.

Duffy Y (1997) Dinosaurs are holding nurses back. Nursing Standard 12(10): 10–11.

Dutton A (1968) Factors Affecting Recruitment of Nurse Tutors. A survey carried out on behalf of the Kings Fund and RCN. London: King Edwards Hospital Fund for London.

Dyson R (1998) Training and pay behind haemorrhage of NHS staff. The Times (Letters to the Editor), 11 August: 17.

Earnshaw C (1997) Too busy studying to give patient care. Nursing Standard (Letters) 12(13–15): 12.

Elkan R, Hillman R, Robinson J (1993) The Implementation of Project 2000 in a District Health Authority: The Effect on the Nursing Service. Nottingham: University of Nottingham.

Emmet DM (1958) Function: Purpose and Powers. London: Macmillan and Co. Ltd.

Emmet DM (1986) Professional ethics. In Macquarrie J, Childress JF, (Eds) A New Dictionary of Christian Ethics. London: SCM Press Ltd. pp 502–4.

ENB (1983) The End of the Beginning. London: ENB.

ENB (1985a) Syllabus and Examinations for Courses in General Nursing Leading to Registration in Part 1 of the Register. Letter 1985 (19) ERDB, April. London: ENB.

ENB (1985b) Professional Education/Training Courses: Consultation Paper. Letter, 14 May. London: ENB.

ENB (1991) Midwifery and Health Visiting. Framework for Continuing Professional Education for Nurses, Midwives and Health Visitors: Guide to Implementation. London: ENB, September.

ENB (1993a) Regulations and Guidelines for the Approval of Institutions and Courses. London: ENB.

ENB (1993b) Guidelines for Educational Audit. London: ENB.

ENB (1994) Creating Lifelong Learners: Guidelines for Pre-registration Nursing Programmes of Education. London: ENB.

ENB (1995) Creating Lifelong Learners, Partnerships for Care: Guidelines for the Implementation of the UKCC's Standards for Education and Practice following Registration. London: ENB. June.

ENB (1996) Regulations and Guidelines for the Approval of Institutions and Programmes. London: ENB. February.

ENB (1997a) Standards for Approval of Higher Education Institutions and Programmes. London: ENB. October.

ENB (1997b) Guidelines for External Examiners. London: ENB. October.

ENB (1997c) Analysis of English National Board for Nursing, Midwifery and Health Visiting Statistics. London: ENB.

ENB (1998a) Response to the Review of the Nurses, Midwives and Health Visitors Act 1997. London: ENB.

ENB (1998b) Annual Report 1997–1998. London: ENB.

ENB (1998c) Quality Assurance Manual. London: ENB.

ENB (2000) Annual Report 1999–2000. London: ENB.

ENB News (1997) Review of the Nurses, Midwives and Health Visitors Act, 1997: progress. ENB News 26: 1.

ENB News (1998a) Review of the Nurses, Midwives and Health Visitors Act 1997. ENB News 27: 1.

ENB News (1998b) Trends in student numbers on pre-registration programmes. ENB News 27: 6.

ENB News (1998c) A Summary of the Board's response to the Review of the Nurses, Midwives and Health Visitors Act 1997. ENB News 28: 1, 12.

ENB News (1999) Board's evidence to UKCC Commission for Education. ENB News 32: 8.

English T (1997) Medicine in the 1990s needs a team approach. British Medical Journal (Education and debate) 314: 661–63.

Eraut M, Alderton J, Boylan A, Wraight A (1995) Learning to Use Scientific Knowledge in Education and Practice Settings: An Evaluation of the Contribution of the Biological, Behavioural and Social Sciences to Pre-registration Nursing and Midwifery Programmes. London: ENB.

Fabricius J (1999) The crisis in nursing: reflections on the crisis. Psychoanalytic Psychotherapy 13(3): 203–6.

Fawkes BN (1970) Recent proposal for developments in nursing education in England and Wales. International Nursing Review 17(3): 258–65.

Fawkes BN (1972) Needs of education and training in nursing. Nursing Times (Occasional papers) 68(18): 69–71.

Fearon M (1998) Assessment and measurement of competence in practice. Nursing Standard 12(22): 43–47.

Felix C (1998) Reflection is not imposed as a punishment . . . it just feels as if has been [sic]. Nursing Times (Letters) 94(12): 23.

Ferriman A (1998) Decline in altruism threatens blood supplies. British Medical Journal (News) 317: 1405.

Finlayson LR, Nazroo JY (1998) Gender Inequalities in Nursing Careers. Report No. 854. London: Policy Studies Institute.

Fisher E (1937) The Nurse's Textbook. London: Faber and Faber Ltd.

Fisher P (1998) Nursing crisis. The Independent (Letters), 29 January: 20.

Fitzpatrick R (1993) Scope and measurement of patient satisfaction. In Fitzpatrick R, Hopkins A, (Eds) Measurement of Patients' Satisfaction with Their Care. London: Royal College of Physicians of London. pp 1–17.

Fleming J (1985) The great escape. Senior Nurse 3(2): 54–55.

Foskett NH, Hemsley-Brown JV (1998) Perceptions of nursing as a career amongst young people in schools and colleges. University of Southampton, Centre for Research in Education and Marketing, Department of Health. March.

Fox EM (1912) Nursing ethics. Nursing Times 8, (366): 475–478, May 4.

Fox EM (1914) First Lines in Nursing. London: The Scientific Press. (2nd edn, 1924; 3rd edn, 1930)

Francis B, Peelo M, Soothill K (1992) NHS nursing, vocation, career or just a job? In Soothill K, Henry C, Kendrick K, (Eds) Themes and Perspectives in Nursing. London: Chapman and Hall. pp 56–74.

Freidson E (1986) Professional Powers. Chicago: The University of Chicago Press.

Gaba M (1997) Don't go changin'. Nursing Standard (Opinion) 11(38): 18.

Gabbitass G (1998) Experience makes a good nurse. Daily Mail (Letters), 24 December: 60.

General Medical Council (1993) Tomorrow's Doctors: Recommendations on Undergraduate Medical Education. London: GMC. December.

George S (1999) Back to the future. Nursing Times 95(1): 62–63.

Gerrish K, McManus M, Ashworth P (1997) The Assessment of Practice at Diploma, Degree and Postgraduate Levels in Nursing and Midwifery Education: Literature Review and Documentary Analysis. London: ENB.

Ghazi F, Henshaw L (1998) How to keep student nurses motivated. Nursing Standard 13(8): 43–48.

Gibberd B (1988) Project 2000 – the only option? The Health Service Journal p. 182–183, February 11.

Gillespie A, Curzio J (1998) Blood pressure measurement: assessing staff knowledge. Nursing Standard 12(23): 35–37.

Gillon R (1986) Nursing ethics and medical ethics. Journal of Medical Ethics (Editorial) 12: 115–16, 122.

Girvin J (1998) Speaking out. Nursing Times 94(20): 21.

Glen J (1997) Nursing is not just about studying. Nursing Standard (Letters) 12(9): 11.

Gloucestershire Community Health Council (1999) In the Patient's Interest: A study of the Management of Nursing in Gloucestershire's Acute Hospitals. Gloucester: Gloucestershire Community Health Council.

GNC (1923a) Syllabus of Lectures and Demonstrations for Education and Training in General Nursing. London: GNC.

GNC (1923b) Syllabus of Subjects for Examination for the Certificate of General Nursing. London: GNC. (Revised 1925, 1933, 1939, 1952, 1955, 1958, 1962)

GNC (1952) Syllabus of Subjects for Examination for the Certificate of General Nursing for Male Nurses. London: GNC.

GNC (1962) Guide to the Syllabus of Subjects for Examination for the Certificate of General Nursing. London: GNC.

GNC (1965) Memorandum on the Platt Report. Nursing Times 61(40): 1347–49.

GNC (1969) Syllabus of Subjects for Examination and Record of Practical Instruction and Experience for the Certificate of General Nursing. London: GNC. (Reprinted 1973, 1974, 1976)

GNC (1977a) Training Syllabus Register of Nurses: General Nursing, Amended 1977. London: GNC.

GNC (1977b) Educational Policy: Policy Statement Applying to all Parts of the Register and Roll: 77/19/A. London: GNC.

GNC (1977c) Educational Policy: Syllabus and Practical Experiences Required for Admission to the General Part of the Register: Revising Council's Circular 69/4/3: 77/19/B. London: GNC.

GNC (1977d) Syllabus of Training: Professional Register – Part 1 (Registered General Nurse), Amended 1977. London: GNC.

GNC (undated) Record of Practical Instruction and Experience for the Certificate of General Nursing. London: GNC.

Godfrey K (1999) First things first. Nursing Times 95(24): 24.

Goldhill DR, Worthington LM, Mulcahy AJ, Tarling MM (1999) Quality of care before admission to intensive care, deaths on the ward might be prevented. British Medical Journal (Letters) 318: 195.

Goodwin L, Bosanquet N (1985) Implications for the costs of nurse training in the UK of changes in learner status. Annexe of Research Studies for Commission on Nursing Education, The Education of Nurses: A New Dispensation. London: RCN. pp. 201–58.

Gott M (1984) Learning Nursing. London: RCN.

Gough P (1998) The future is yours. Nursing Times (Insight) 94(26): 30–32.

Gould D, Chamberlain A (1997) The use of a ward-based educational teaching package to enhance nurses' compliance with infection control procedures. Journal of Clinical Nursing 6: 55–67.

Gould M (1998) Learning the script. Nursing Standard (News analysis) 12(25): 14.

Gration HM (1944) The Practice of Nursing London: Faber and Faber Ltd. (2nd edn, 1946)

Gration HM, Holland DL (1950) The Practice of Nursing. 3rd edn. London: Faber and Faber Ltd. (4th edn, 1954; 5th edn, 1956; 6th edn, 1959)

Guardian (1996) Worry grows over nurses. The Guardian, 5 September: 9.

Guardian (1998) Nurses' paperwork cuts time for patient care. The Guardian, 5 August: 5.

Guardian (1999a) Labour admits NHS crisis. The Guardian, 9 January: 1.

Guardian (1999b) Reform of nursing watchdog "will offer greater degree of protection". The Guardian, 9 February: 5.

Guardian (1999c) Shake-up to give trainee nurses more ward skills. The Guardian, 11 September: 9.

Guardian (1999d) Nurses set for return to practical skills. The Guardian, 22 November: 10.

Gulland A, O'Dowd A (1999) Pressure gauge. Nursing Times 95(42): 14–15.

Hadley WJ (1902) Nursing: General, Medical and Surgical London: J and A Churchill. (2nd edn, 1907)

Hallam J (2000) Nursing the Image. London: Routledge.

Handy C (1984) The Future of Work. Oxford: Robertson.

Handy C (1989) The Age of Unreason. London: Hutchinson.

Handy C (1998) The Hungry Spirit. London: Arrow Books Ltd.

Harding-Price D (1997) Practice-based skills come first. Nursing Standard (Letters) 12(9): 11.

Harper M (1998) Nursing degree. The Scotsman (Letters to the Editor), 14 August: 14.

Harris M (1999) Degrees that signal the end of real nurses. The Express (Comment), 13 January.

Hay R (1994) A nurse's place . . . is at the bedside. Nursing Standard (Viewpoint) 8(27): 42–43.

Health Act (1999) Chapter 8. London: The Stationary Office.

Health Act, Explanatory Notes (1999) Chapter 8. London: The Stationary Office.

Health Advisory Service 2000 (1998) Not Because they are Old. London: Department of Health, NHSE.

Health Service Commissioner for England, for Scotland and for Wales (1995) Third Report for Session 1994–95: Annual Report for 1994–95. London: HMSO.

Health Service Commissioner for England, for Scotland and for Wales (1997) First Report for Session 1997–8: Annual Report for 1996–97, HC41. London: The Stationery Office.

Health Service Commissioner for England, for Scotland and for Wales (1998) Investigations Completed April–September 1998: 1st Report – Session 1998–99, HC3. London: The Stationery Office.

Hector W (1972) The role and preparation of the teacher. Nursing Times 68(46): 1460–61.

Hek G (1994) Adding up the cost of teaching mathematics. Nursing Standard 8(22): 25–29.

Help the Aged (1999a) The Views of Older People on Hospital Care: A Survey, January 1999. London: Help the Aged.

Help the Aged (1999b) Dignity on the Ward – A Campaign Update – October 1999. London: Help the Aged.

Help the Aged (1999c) Failing Older People – Flaws in the NHS Complaints Procedure. London: Help the Aged.

Henwood M (1998) Ignored and Invisible? Carers' experience of the NHS. London: Carers National Association.

Her Majesty's Government (1997) The New NHS, Modern, Dependable (White Paper), Cmd 3807. London: The Stationery Office.

Hewison J (1998) Angels on the verge of despair. The Times Higher Education Supplement, 31 July: 14–15.

Hewison J, Millar B, Dowswell T (1998a) Changing Patterns of Training Provision: Implications for Access and Equity: Full Report of Research Activities and Results. Swindon: Economic and Social Research Council, University of Leeds.

Hewison J, Millar B, Dowswell T (1998b) Changing Patterns of Training Provision: Implications for Access and Equity: Summary of Research Results. Swindon: Economic and Social Research Council, University of Leeds.

Higgins R, Hurst K, Wistow G (1998) The Mental Health Nursing Care Provided for Acute Psychiatric Patients. Research Bulletin, Department of Health and Nuffield Institute for Health, June.

Hinde J (1998) Nurses are not carrying on. The Times Higher Education Supplement, 27 November: 6-7.

Hobbs R, Murray ET (1999) Specialist liaison nurses. British Medical Journal (Editorial) 218: 683–84.

HoC (1978a) Nurses, Midwives and Health Visitors Bill. House of Commons Official Report. Parliamentary Debates (Hansard), 2 November, vol 957, col 200–32. London: HMSO.

HoC (1978b) Nurses, Midwives and Health Visitors Bill. House of Commons Official Report. Parliamentary Debates (Hansard), 13 November, vol 958, col 35–126. London: HMSO.

HoC (1978c) Nurses, Midwives and Health Visitors Bill. House of Commons Official Report. Parliamentary Debates. Standing Committee B, 28, 30 November, 5, 7, 12, 14 December, vol I. London: HMSO.

HoC (1979a) Nurses, Midwives and Health Visitors Bill. House of Commons Official Report. Parliamentary Debates. Standing Committee B, 18, 23 January, vol I. London: HMSO.

HoC (1979b) Nurses, Midwives and Health Visitors Bill. House of Commons Official Report. Parliamentary Debates (Hansard), 7 February, vol 962, col 413–509. London: HMSO.

HoC (1992a) Nurses, Midwives and Health Visitors Bill. House of Commons Official Report. Parliamentary Debates (Hansard), 13 January, vol 201, col 696–722. London: HMSO.

HoC (1992b) Nurses, Midwives and Health Visitors Bill. House of Commons Official Report. Parliamentary Debates. Standing Committee B, 28, 29, 30 January, vol II. London: HMSO.

HoC (1992c) Nurses, Midwives and Health Visitors Bill. House of Commons Official Report. Parliamentary Debates (Hansard), 4 March, vol 205, col 387–98. London: HMSO.

HoC (1997) Nurses, Midwives and Health Visitors Act. (Written answers) House of Commons Offical Report. Parliamentary Debates (Hansard), 13 March, vol 292, col 345. London: The Stationary Office.

HoC (1998a) Relationship between Health and Social Services. House of Commons Health Committee, Minutes of Evidence, Wednesday 25 February, Session 1997–98. London: The Stationery Office.

HoC (1998b) National Health Service. House of Commons Official Report. Parliamentary Debates (Hansard), 9 July, vol. 315, col 1246–1337. London: The Stationary Office.

HoC (1998c) Report of the Health Service Ombudsman for 1996–1997 Select Committee on Public Administration Second Report: Report together with the Proceedings of the Committee and Minutes of Evidence, Session 1997–1998, (HC 352). London: The Stationery Office.

HoC (1999a) National Health Service. House of Commons Official Report. Parliamentary Debates (Hansard), 11 January, vol 323, col 35–54. London: The Stationery Office.

HoC (1999b) Nursing Care (Eastbourne Hospital). House of Commons Official Report. Parliamentary Debates (Hansard), 24 May, vol. 332, col 134–42. London: The Stationary Office

HoC (1999c) Opposition Day Debate, Health Care. House of Commons Official Report. Parliamentary Debates (Hansard), 20 July, vol. 335, col 974–1032. London: The Stationery Office.

HoC (1999d) Nurse Training. Written Answers. House of Commons Official Report. Parliamentary Debates (Hansard), 27 July, vol 336, col 236. London: The Stationery Office.

HoC (1999e) Future NHS Staffing requirements, Third Report (Vol. I), Report and Proceedings of the Committee, Session 1998–1999. House of Commons Health Committee. London: The Stationery Office.

HoC (1999f) Procedures Related to Adverse Clinical Incidents and Outcomes in Medical Care, Sixth Report (Vol. I), Report and Proceedings of the Committee. House of Commons Health Committee. London: The Stationery Office.

HoC (1999g) Procedures Related to Adverse Clinical Incidents and Outcomes in Medical Care, Sixth Report (Vol. II), Minutes of Evidence and Appendices. House of Commons Health Committee. London: The Stationery Office.

HoC (1999h) Long-term care. House of Commons Official Report. Parliamentary Debates (Hansard), 2 December, vol 340, col 444–530. London: The Stationery Office.

HoC (2000) The Management and Control of Hospital Acquired Infections in Acute NHS Trusts in England. Select Committee on Public Accounts. Forty Second Report. London: The Stationary Office.

HoL (1890) Report of the Select Committee of the House of Lords on Metropolitan Hospitals with Minutes of Evidence, appendix and index. vol. xvi, London: HMSO.

HoL (1891) Second Report of the Select Committee of the House of Lords on Metropolitan Hospitals with Minutes of Evidence, appendix and index. vol. xvi, London: HMSO.

HoL (1978) Queen's Speech. House of Lords Official Report. Parliamentary Debates (Hansard), 1 November, vol 396, col 1-7. London: HMSO.

HoL (1979a) Nurses, Midwives and Health Visitors Bill. House of Lords Official Report. Parliamentary Debates (Hansard), 12 February, vol 398, col 1086. London: HMSO.

HoL (1979b) Nurses, Midwives and Health Visitors Bill. House of Lords Official Report. Parliamentary Debates (Hansard), 19 February, vol 398, col 1643–81. London: HMSO.

HoL (1979c) Nurses, Midwives and Health Visitors Bill. House of Lords Official Report. Parliamentary Debates (Hansard), 13 March, vol 399, col 504–57. London: HMSO.

HoL (1979d) Nurses, Midwives and Health Visitors Bill. House of Lords Official Report. Parliamentary Debates (Hansard), 27 March, vol 399, col 1473–96. London: HMSO.

HoL (1979e) Nurses, Midwives and Health Visitors Bill. House of Lords Official Report. Parliamentary Debates (Hansard), 2 April, vol 399, col 1726–29. London: HMSO.

HoL (1979f) Nurses, Midwives and Health Visitors Bill. House of Lords Official Report. Parliamentary Debates (Hansard), 4 April, vol 399, col 1953–54. London: HMSO.

HoL (1991a) Nurses, Midwives and Health Visitors Bill. House of Lords Official Report. Parliamentary Debates (Hansard), 12 November, vol 532, col 482–86, 492–508. London: HMSO.

HoL (1991b) Nurses, Midwives and Health Visitors Bill. House of Lords Official Report. Parliamentary Debates (Hansard), 26 November, vol 532, col 1277–99. London: HMSO.

HoL (1991c) Nurses, Midwives and Health Visitors Bill. House of Lords Official Report. Parliamentary Debates (Hansard), 9 December, vol 533, col 523–33. London: HMSO.

HoL (1998a) Nurses in the NHS. House of Lords Official Report. Parliamentary Debates (Hansard), 16 June, vol. 590, col 1539–66. London: The Stationery Office.

HoL (1998b) Written answers (Lord Stoddart of Swindon, Baroness Jay), NHS, Treatment of "Customers". House of Lords Official Report. Parliamentary Debates (Hansard), 30 June, vol 591, col 75. London: The Stationery Office.

HoL (1998c) Written answers, (Lord Stoddart of Swindon, Baroness Jay), Patients' Charter, use of Christian names. House of Lords Official Report. Parliamentary Debates (Hansard), 8 July, vol 591, col 143. London: The Stationery Office.

HoL (1999a) Health Bill. House of Lords Official Report. Parliamentary Debates (Hansard), 9 February, vol. 597, col 107–88. London: The Stationery Office.

HoL (1999b) Care Standards Bill – Second Reading, Parliamentary Debates (Hansard), December 13, vol. 608, No. 15. c. 34–80. London: The Stationery Office.

HoL (1999c) Elderly patients: NHS hospital treatment, Parliamentary Debates (Hansard), December 15, vol. 608, No. 17, c. 217–219.

HoL (2000a) Motion – Nurse education and practice. House of Lords Official Report. Parliamentary Debates (Hansard), 26 January, vol 608, col 1556–1695. London: The Stationery Office.

HoL (2000b) Motion – National Health Service. House of Lords Official Report. Parliamentary Debates (Hansard), 2 February, vol 609, col 237–316. London: The Stationery Office.

Horton R (1997) Health: A complicated game of doctors and nurses. The Observer (Life: Mind and Body), 30 March: 53.

Houghton M (1938) Aids to Practical Nursing. London: Baillière, Tindall and Cox. (2nd edn, 1940; 3rd edn, 1941; 4th edn, 1942; 5th edn, 1947; 6th edn, 1948; 7th edn, 1952; 8th edn, 1956; 9th edn, 1960)

Huehns T (1988) 'The nurses are wonderful but what are these pills for?' Geriatric Medicine, June: 45–50.

Humphry L (1889) A Manual of Nursing: Medical and Surgical. London: Charles Griffin and Company Limited.

Hutt R, Connor H, Hirsh W (1985) The Manpower Implications of Possible Changes in Basic Nurse Training: A Report for the RCN's Commission on Nursing Education. Brighton: Institute of Manpower Studies, University of Sussex.

Incomes Data Services Ltd (1997) Public sector labour market survey 1997. IDS Report 751. London: IDS. pp 25–32.

Incomes Data Services Ltd (1998) Public sector labour market 1998. IDS Report 775. London: IDS. pp 10–23. December.

Incomes Data Services Ltd (1999) Public sector labour market survey. IDS Report 799. London: IDS. pp 10–19. December.

Incomes Data Services Ltd. (2000) NHS health care assistants. IDS Report: pay, Conditions and Labour Market Changes, 819: 8, October.

Independent (1999) Nurses' leaders warn 15,000 vacancies need to be filled. The Independent, 19 October: 8.

Jacka K, Lewin D (1987) The Clinical Learning of Student Nurses. NERU Report Number 6. London: Nursing Education Research Unit, University of London.

James P, Day H (1997) Education is just part of holistic nursing. Nursing Standard (Letters) 12(13–15): 12.

Jenkins S (1998) Why I left the NHS after 26 years. Nursing Standard (Letters) 12(49): 10.

Jenkinson T (1999) Project 2000, no return to a mythical "golden age". Nursing Times (Letters) 95(42): 20.

JM Consulting Ltd (1998a) The Regulation of Nurses, Midwives and Health Visitors: Invitation to Comment on Issues Raised by a Review of the Nurses, Midwives and Health Visitors Act 1997. Bristol: JM Consulting Ltd. January.

JM Consulting Ltd (1998b) The Regulation of Nurses, Midwives and Health Visitors: Report on a Review of the Nurses, Midwives and Health Visitors Act 1997. Bristol: JM Consulting Ltd. August.

Jones L, Leneman L, Maclean U (1987) Consumer Feedback for the NHS: A Literature Review. London: King Edwards Hospital Fund for London.

Jordan S, Potter N (1999) Biosciences on the margin. Nursing Standard 13(25): 46–48.

Jowett S, Walton I, Payne S (1994) Challenges and Change in Nurse Education – A Study of the Implementation of Project 2000. Slough: NFER.

Judge H (1986) A college education? Nursing Times, 82(29): 31–2.

Katz FE (1969) Nurses. In Etzioni A (Ed) The Semi-professions and Their Organization. New York: The Free Press. pp 54–81.

King E (1998) Nurses won't get hands-on. Daily Express (Letters to the Editor), 11 August 11: 9.

Kitson AL (1996) Does nursing have a future? British Medical Journal 313: 1647–51.

Kratz C (1986) Thoughts on the project. Nursing Times 82(42): 55.

Lask S, Smith P, Masterson A (1994) A Curricular Review of the Pre-and Post-Registration Education Programmes for Nurses, Midwives and Health Visitors in Relation to the Integration of a Philosophy of Health: Developing a Model for Evaluation. London: ENB.

Latter S, Yerrell P, Rycroft-Malone J, Shaw D (2000) Nursing and Medication Education: Concept Analysis Research for Curriculum and Practice Development. London: English National Board for Nursing, Midwifery and Health Visiting.

Lawson N (1996) Is it the end for nurses? The Times, 26 December: 17.

Lawson N (1999) Nurses deserve to be paid for their skills. The Observer, 17 January: 30.

Le Fanu J (1995) Nurse, put on your uniform. The Sunday Telegraph (Review) 20 August: 2.

Le Grand J (1997) Knights, knaves or pawns? Human behaviour and social policy. Journal of Social Policy 26(2): 149–69.

Lees FS (1874) Handbook for Hospital Sisters. (Ed: Acland HW) London: WS Isbister and Co.

Lelean SR (1975) Ready for Report Nurse? London: RCN.

Lewis PG (1890) Nursing: Its Theory and Practice. London: The Scientific Press, Ltd. (2nd edn, 1891; 3rd edn, 1892; 4th edn, 1893; 8th edn, 1895; 11th edn, 1899)

Lilley R (1999) Nursing shortage and NHS decline. The Times (Letters to the Editor), 12 January: 17.

Lipley N (1998) Peach of a job. Nursing Standard 12(47): 14.

Longhurst RH (1998a) Down in the mouth. Nursing Times 94(46): 24–25.

Longhurst RH (1998b) A cross-sectional study of the oral health care instruction given to nurses during their basic training. British Dental Journal 184(9): 453–57.

Lord Stoddart of Swindon (1998) Personal communication to Ann Bradshaw, 6 August.

Lückes ECE (1892) Lectures on General Nursing. London: Kegan Paul, Trench, Trübner and Co, Ltd. (4th edn, 1898)

Luker KA, Hogg C, Austin L, Ferguson B, Smith K (1998) Decision making, the context of nurse prescribing. Journal of Advanced Nursing 27: 657–65.

Luker K, Carlisle C, Riley E, Stilwell J, Davies C, Wilson R (1997) Project 2000 Fitness for Purpose: Report to the Department of Health, December 1996. University of Warwick, Centre for Health Services Studies, Institute for Employment Research; University of Liverpool, Department of Nursing Studies.

MacGuire J (1961) From Student to Nurse – The Induction Period: A Study of Student Nurses in the First Six Months of Training in Five Schools of Nursing. Oxford: Oxford Area Nurse Training Committee. September.

MacGuire J (1966) From Student to Nurse – Training and Qualification: A Study of Student Nurses in Training at Five Schools of Nursing. Oxford: Oxford Area Nurse Training Committee. May.

Mackay L (1989) Nursing a Problem. Milton Keynes: Open University Press.

Mackay L (1998) Nursing, will the idea of vocation survive?. In Abbott P, Meerabeau L (Eds) The Sociology of the Caring Professions. London: UCL Press. pp 54–72.

Macleod Clark J, Maben J, Jones K (1996) Project 2000: Perceptions of the Philosophy and Practice of Nursing. London: ENB.

Marrin M (1999) Nurses are the problem. Sunday Telegraph, 10 January: 31.

Marsh DC, Willcocks AJ (1965) Focus on Nurse Recruitment: A Snapshot from the Provinces. London: OUP, published for the Nuffield Provincial Hospitals Trust.

May N, Veitch L, McIntosh JB, Alexander MF (1997) Preparation for Practice: Evaluation of Nurse and Midwife Education in Scotland 1992 Programmes: Final Report. Glasgow: Glasgow Caledonian University.

May P (1999) The crisis in the nursing profession: should we bring back ward sisters? Church of England Newspaper, 10 December: 16.

Maynard A (2000) Bleating up the wrong tree. Health Service Journal 110(5734): 18–19.

McFarlane J (1985) Contemporary challenges in education for the caring professions, education for nursing, midwifery, and health visiting. British Medical Journal 291: 268–71.

McFarlane J, Castledine G (1982) A Guide to the Practice of Nursing Using the Nursing Process. London: The CV Mosby Company.

McManus IC, Richards P, Winder BC, Sproston KA (1998) Clinical experience, performance in final examination and learning style in medical students, prospective study: British Medical Journal 316: 345–50.

Meadows S, Levenson R, Baeza J (2000) The Last Straw: Explaining the NHS Nursing Shortage. London: King's Fund.

Medical Devices Agency (1995a) The Report of the Expert Working Group on Alarms on Clinical Monitors. London: Department of Health.

Medical Devices Agency (1995b) Infusions Systems: Device bulletin MDA DB9503. London: Department of Health.

Mencap (1998) The NHS – Health for all? London: Mencap.

Menzies IEP (1960) A case study in the functioning of social systems as a defence against anxiety: a report on a study of the nursing service of a general hospital. Human Relations 13: 95–121.

Menzies IEP (1961a) Nurses under stress – 1. Nursing Times 57(5): 141–42.

Menzies IEP (1961b) Nurses under stress – 2. Nursing Times 57(6): 173–74.

Menzies IEP (1961c) Nurses under stress – 3. Nursing Times 57(7): 206–8.

Menzies IEP (1970) A Case Study in the Functioning of Social Systems as a Defence against Anxiety: A Report on a Study of the Nursing Service of a General

Hospital: (Reprint of Tavistock Pamplet No. 3). London: Tavistock Institute of Human Relations.

Menzies-Lyth I (1999) The crisis in nursing: Facing the crisis. Psychoanalytic Psychotherapy 13(3): 2207–12.

Mercator (1997) Nursing Standard 'Lifestyle' Survey, SNP12015. Harrow: Nursing Standard.

Meredith P, Wood C (1997) The Patient's Experience of Surgery: A Selective Evaluation of Two Hospital Sites. London: Patient Satisfaction with Surgery Audit Service, Royal College of Surgeons. August.

Milburn A (1999) Key speech: Making a difference: Nursing and midwifery education. Keynote speech by Secretary of State. London, 22 November.

Milburn A (2000) Key speech: RCN Annual Congress. London, 5 April.

Mills M (1998) Back to basics. The Daily Telegraph (Letters to the Editor), 10 August: 19.

Ministry of Health Scottish Home and Health Department (1966) Report of the Committee on Senior Nursing Staff. Chairman, Brian Salmon. London: HMSO.

Mitchell JRA (1984a) Is nursing any business of doctors? A simple guide to the "nursing process". British Medical Journal 288: 216–19.

Mitchell Tony (1984b) The nursing process debate, is nursing any business of doctors? Nursing Times 80(19): 28–32.

Moore J (1988) Letter from the Secretary of State, DHSS, to Miss Audrey Emerton, Chairman of the UKCC, 20 May.

Moores Y, Deegan M (1997) Letter from Chief Nursing Officer/Director of Nursing and Deputy Director of Human Resources to Trust Nurse Executive Directors, Members of Education Consortia, Heads of Faculties and Departments Providing Pre-Registration Nurse Education; Copy to Regional Education and Development Groups, Regional Office Education Leads, UKCC, ENB. Project 2000 – Fitness for Purpose: A Report of Research Undertaken for the Department of Health by the Universities of Warwick and Liverpool. Quarry Hill, Leeds: NHSE Headquarters. September.

Morgan O (1998) Who Cares? The Great British Health Debate. Abingdon: Radcliffe Medical Press.

Moroney J (1950) Surgery for Nurses. Edinburgh: E and S Livingstone. (2nd edn, 1952; 3rd edn, 1955; 4th edn, 1956; 5th edn, 1958; 6th edn, 1959; 7th edn, 1961; 8th edn, 1962; 9th edn, 1964; 10th edn, 1966; 11th edn, 1967; 12th edn, 1971; 13th edn, 1975; 14th edn, 1978; 15th edn, 1982)

Morris A (1997) Unnerved by the push for degrees. Nursing Standard 12(11): 11.

Morton-Williams J, Berthoud R (1971a) Nurses Attitude Study: Report on Depth Interviews. (Ref. 02.194) London: Social and Community Planning Research. February.

Morton-Williams J, Berthoud R (1971b) Nurses Attitude Survey. (Ref. 02.188) London: Social and Community Planning Research. November.

Munro R (1999) Could do better. Nursing Times 95(1): 60–62.

Murray T (1997) If all nurses are graduates duties will be passed on. Nursing Standard (Letters) 12(12): 10.

National Audit Office (1992) Nursing Education: Implementation of Project 2000 in England. Report by the Comptroller and Auditor General. London: HMSO. 4 December.

National Audit Office (2000) The Management and Control of Hospital Acquired Infection in Acute NHS Trusts in England. Report by the Comptroller and Auditor General. London: The Stationary Office, HC 230 Session 1998–00. 17 February.

National Committee of Inquiry into Higher Education (1997) Higher Education in the Learning Society: Report of the National Committee. Chairman, Sir Ron Dearing. Crown Copyright, July.

National Consumer Council (1999) Self-regulation of Professionals in Health Care: Consumer Issues. PD35/H/99. London: National Consumer Council. June.

Neary M (1999) Preparing assessors for continuous assessment. Nursing Standard 13(18): 41–47.

Nessling RC (1989) The Professional Nursing Labour Market: Developing a Regional Perspective. North West Thames Regional Health Authority, Nursing Department. 12 December.

Newton G (1998) Workforce costs. Nursing Times 94(3): 62.

NHSE (1998a) A Consultation on a Strategy for Nursing, Midwifery and Health Visiting. Health Service Circular HSC, 1998/045. London: Department of Health, NHSE. 20 April.

NHSE (1998b) A First Class Service: Quality in the New NHS. York: NHSE.

NHSE (1998c) Evaluation of the Pilot Project Programme of Children with Life-threatening Illnesses. York: NHSE.

NHSE (1998d) Nurse Consultants. Health Service Circular HSC, 1998/161. London: Department of Health, NHSE. 22 September.

NHSE (1999a) Review of the Nurses, Midwives and Health Visitors Act: Government Response to the Recommendations. Health Service Circular HSC 1999/030. London: Department of Health, NHSE. 9 February.

NHSE (1999b) Making a Difference to Nursing and Midwifery Pre-Registration Education. Health Service Circular HSC 1999/219. London: Department of Health, NHSE. 27 September.

NHSE (2000) Outcomes for the End of Year 1 of the Pre-registration Nurse Education Programme. Leeds: NHSE. February.

NHSE South East (1999) Report of the Review of Nursing at Eastbourne Hospitals NHS Trust. Greenwood R (Chair). NHSE South East.

Nicklin P, Kenworthy N (1995) Teaching and Assessing in Nursing Practice: An Experiential Approach. London: Scutari Press.

Nightingale F (1888) Letters and addresses to the Probationer Nurses in the Nightingale Fund School at St Thomas's Hospital and Nurses who were formerly trained there. Original letters and prints for private circulation held by University College, London. 16 May.

Nurses Midwives and Health Visitors Act (1979) London: HMSO.

Nursing Standard (1997a) Editorial. Nursing Standard 11(16): 1.

Nursing Standard (1997b) UKCC will deal with incompetent practice. Nursing Standard 11(26): 9.

Nursing Standard (1997c) Science vs art (readers panel). Credibility counts but only at the right level (Carol Singleton). Academia cannot make a good nurse (Steve Flatt). Without hands-on nurses what would researchers do? (Stephen Weeks). Nursing Standard 11(39): 19.

Nursing Standard (1997d) UKCC figures show crisis is worsening. Worrying decline in student applicants. Nursing Standard 12(9): 5.

Nursing Standard (1998a) Emphasis on challenge of nursing in £12 million recruitment drive. Nursing Standard 12(16): 5.

Nursing Standard (1998b) UKCC holds closed session on regulation. Nursing Standard 12(24): 5.

Nursing Standard (1998c) NDU effect on patient not known. Nursing Standard 12(24): 9.

Nursing Standard (1998d) DoH holds back new figures on shortages. Nursing Standard 12(26): 5.

Nursing Standard (1998e) DoH figures confirm recruitment crisis. Nursing Standard 12(30): 6.

Nursing Standard (1998f) Most complaints to UKCC are trivial or not appropriate. Nursing Standard 12(37): 5.

Nursing Standard (1998g) Expanded role needs funding. Nursing Standard 12(38): 6.

Nursing Standard (1998h) 80,000 to be surveyed for review of education 12(38): 6.

Nursing Standard (1998i) Figures show decline in nursing applicants. Nursing Standard 12(39): 7.

Nursing Standard (1998j) Increase numbers of nurses not doctors. Nursing Standard 12(42): 7.

Nursing Standard (1998k) Male nurses make up half of misconduct cases. Nursing Standard 12(48): 5.

Nursing Standard (1998l) UKCC promotes message that PREP is very simple. Nursing Standard 12(48): 6.

Nursing Standard (1998m) Blair announces five point plan for nursing. Nursing Standard 12(51): 5.

Nursing Standard (1999a) Nurses are "detached" and not interested in PREP. Nursing Standard 13(24): 7.

Nursing Standard (1999b) Clark launches attack on England's nursing strategy. Nursing Standard 13(47).

Nursing Standard (1999c) UKCC education review supports Project 2000. Nursing Standard 13(52): 4–5.

Nursing Standard (1999d) December deadline for education action plans. Nursing Standard 14(2): 6.

Nursing Standard (1999e) UKCC figures reveal downturn in registered nurses. 14(6): 5.

Nursing Standard (1999f) Recruitment crisis easing, says minister. Nursing Standard 14(9): 5.

Nursing Standard (1999g) Pilot project will regrade nurses and junior doctors. Ministers to rethink roles of health professionals. Nursing Standard 14(10): 5.

Nursing Standard (2000a) Nurses to set standards for better hospital care. Nursing Standard 14(20): 5.

Nursing Standard (2000b) Patients more likely to complain. Nursing Standard 14(41): 5.

Nursing Standard (2000c) More students on nursing and midwifery courses. Nursing Standard 14(47): 4.

Nursing Standard (2000d) Complaints to UKCC soar. Nursing Standard 14(47): 5.

Nursing Standard (2000e) Government wants regional pay boost to curb shortages. Nursing Standard 15(1): 4.

Nursing Times (1963) The bedpan round. Nursing Times (Editorial) 59(10): 281.

Nursing Times (1972) Bendall on Briggs. Nursing Times, 9 November: 1403.

Nursing Times (1994) UKCC denies sacking as Ralph loses top job. Nursing Times 90(45): 5.

Nursing Times (1997a) UKCC accepts the case for graduate entry. Nursing Times 93(8): 9.

Nursing Times (1997b) UKCC to tackle incompetence. Nursing Times 93(12): 7.

Nursing Times (1997c) Doctor questions nursing care Nursing Times 93(20): 9.

Nursing Times (1997d) Crackdown on incompetence. Nursing Times 93(24): 6.

Nursing Times (1997e) Upsurge in number of complaints to ombudsman. Nurses under fire from ombudsman. Nursing Times 93(50): 9, 17.

Nursing Times (1998a) Nurses deserve a substantial pay award to make up for years of underpayment. Nursing Times (Comment) 94(4): 3.

Nursing Times (1998b) ENB angrily rejects proposed loss of control over courses. Nursing Times 94(9): 6.

Nursing Times (1998c) UKCC plans inquiry into the future of nurse education. Nursing Times 94(10): 6.

Nursing Times (1998d) Nurses could take on police surgeons' work. Nursing Times 94(10): 9.

Nursing Times (1998e) Care assistants to replace nurses in trust budget cuts. Nursing Times 94(23): 6.

Nursing Times (1998f) Staff shortages may wreck Dobson's waiting-list drive. Nursing Times 94(23): 7.

Nursing Times (1998g) Students see nursing as poor prospect. Nursing Times 94(24): 5.

Nursing Times (1998h) UKCC tells nurses to cut out the jargon ASAP. Nursing Times 94(33): 8.

Nursing Times (1999a) UKCC and national boards to be axed. Nursing Times 95(6): 5.

Nursing Times (1999b) Race to sign up. Nursing Times 95(34): 5.

Nursing Times (1999c) UKCC survey uncovers a lack of hands-on training. Nursing Times 95(34): 9.

Nursing Times (1999d) Nursing back in fashion with the nation's students. Nursing Times 95(36): 6.

Nursing Times (1999e) Education leads back to basics. Nursing Times 95(37): 5.

Nursing Times (1999f) Role changes can lead to sloppiness. Nursing Times 95(39): 6.

Nursing Times (1999g) Education reforms "too fast". Nursing Times 95(40): 5.

Nursing Times (1999h) CNO gives a lesson in nursing education. Nursing Times 95(46): 6.

Nursing Times (1999i) Skills shake-up announced. Nursing Times 95(47): 5.

Nursing Times (2000a) Caring, hardworking and maybe a bit bossy. Nursing Times 96(2): 16.

Nursing Times (2000b) Nurse numbers are up, figures out this week show. Nursing Times 96(31): 4.

Nursing Times (2000c) Education chiefs to probe soaring drop-out rates . . . but admissions hit all-time high. Nursing Times 96(36): 6.

Nursing Times (2000d) Nurse vacancies outstrip recruitment. Nursing Times 96(38): 5.

O'Dowd A (1998) Nurse training fails oral exam. Nursing Times 94(46): 25.

Ogden J (1993) Behind closed doors. Nursing Times 89(48): 16.

Oxford Mail (1998) Infusion of cash. Oxford Mail (Voice of the Oxford Mail), 5 June: 8.

Oxford Mail (1998) Patients are dying on JR waiting list. Oxford Mail, 5 June: 1, 3.

Oxford MN (1900) A Handbook of Nursing. London: Methuen and Co Ltd. (2nd edn, 1903; 3rd edn, 1906; 4th edn, 1907; 5th edn, 1909; 6th edn, 1912; 7th edn, 1916; 8th edn, 1923)

Oxford Times (1998) Nurses from Australia to ease crisis. Oxford Times, 12 June: 1.

Oxford Times (1998) Patients dying in hospital crisis. Oxford Times, 12 June: 8.

Parry-Jones WLl (1971) Human relations training in the general hospital. International Journal of Nursing Studies 8: 153–62.

Pearce EC (1937) A General Textbook of Nursing. London Faber and Faber Ltd. (2nd edn, 1938; 3rd edn, 1939; 4th edn, 1940; 5th edn, 1941; 6th edn, 1942; 7th edn, 1942; 8th edn, 1943; 9th edn, 1945; 10th edn, 1959; 11th edn, 1950; 12th edn, 1952; 13th edn, 1953; 14th edn, 1956; 15th edn, 1960; 16th edn, 1963; 17th edn, 1967; 18th edn, 1971)

Pearce EC (1953) Nurse and Patient. London: Faber and Faber Ltd. (2nd edn, 1963; 3rd edn, 1969)

Peelo M, Francis B, Soothill K (1996) NHS nursing, vocation, career or just a job? In Soothill K, Henry C, Kendrick K, (Eds) Themes and Perspectives in Nursing. London: Chapman and Hall, 2nd edn. pp 14–31.

Phillips M (1999a) How the college girls destroyed nursing. Sunday Times, 10 January: 13.

Phillips M (1999b) The real scandal behind this crisis. Daily Mail, 12 January: 8.

Phillips T, Schostak J, Bedford H, Leamon, J (1996) The Evaluation of Pre-Registration Undergraduate Degrees in Nursing and Midwifery (The Tyde Project). London: ENB.

Phillips T, Schostak J, Tyler J, Allen L (2000) Practice and Assessment: An evaluation of the assessment of practice at diploma, degree and postgraduate level in pre- and post-registration nursing and midwifery education. Research Highlights (43) London: English National Board for Nursing, Midwifery and Health Visiting.

Poulton K (1985) The dynamics of change. Senior Nurse 3(5): 13–16.

Price Waterhouse (1988) Nurse Retention and Recruitment: Report on the Factors Affecting the Retention and Recruitment of Nurses, Midwives and Health

Visitors in the NHS. Commissioned by Chairman of Regional Health Authorities in England, Health Boards in Scotland, and Health Authorities in Wales.

Purdy R (1998) Why do we do it? Nursing Standard (Opinion) 12(33): 19.

Ralph C (1993) Regulation and the empowerment of nursing. International Nursing Review 40(2): 58–61.

Raven K (1997) Nursing with a human face. Nursing Standard 12(1): 26.

RCN (1964) A Reform of Nursing Education: First Report of a Special Committee on Nurse Education. Chairman, Sir Harry Platt. London: RCN.

RCN (1971) RCN Evidence to the Committee on Nursing. London: RCN.

RCN (1981a) A Structure for Nursing. London: RCN.

RCN (1981b) Towards Standards: A Discussion Document. London: RCN.

RCN (1985a) The Education of Nurses: A New Dispensation. Commission on Nursing Education. Chairman, Dr Harry Judge. London: RCN.

RCN (1985b) Annexe of Research Studies for Commission on Nursing Education, The Education of Nurses: A New Dispensation. London: RCN.

RCN (1986) Comments on the UKCC's Project 2000 proposals. London: RCN.

RCN (1997a) Oral evidence to pay review body. Intercom 1140: 2–3.

RCN (1997b) Ward Leadership Project: A Journey to Patient-centred Leadership: Executive Summary. London: RCN.

RCN (1997c) Shaping the Future of Nursing Education: A Discussion Document. London: RCN.

RCN (1998a) Review of the Nurses, Midwives and Health Visitors Act, 1997: Response of the RCN. London: RCN. March.

RCN (1998b) Imagining the Future: Nursing in the New Millennium – A Summary Report of the Views of Nurses Involved in the RCN Futures Project. London: RCN.

RCN (1999a) Nurse shortages rising – new figures from Royal College of Nursing reveal. RCN (Press release), 11 January.

RCN (1999b) RCN comment on accusations of involuntary euthanasia in the NHS. RCN (Press release), 7 December.

RCN (2000a) Royal College of Nursing/MORI poll fuels debate around definition of nursing care. RCN (Press release), 13 September.

RCN (2000b) Making up the Difference: A Review of the UK Nursing Labour Market in 2000. Review prepared by the Queen Margaret University College, Edinburgh for the Royal College of Nursing, December.

RCN Employment Information and Research Unit (1998) Employment Brief 18/98: Towards an Inclusive Framework for Multi-skilling: A Discussion Paper. London: RCN.

Redfern S, Norman I, Murrells T, Christian S, Gilmore A, Normand C, Stevens W, Langham S (1997) External Review of the Department of Health-funded Nursing Development Units. London: Kings College, Nursing Research Unit. December.

Registrar's Letter (1993) The Council's Position Concerning a Period of Support and Preceptorship: Implementation of the Post-registration Education and Practice Project (PREPP), Proposals and Annexe. (1/1993, 4 January) London: UKCC.

Registrar's Letter (1995) The Council's Position Concerning a Period of Support and Preceptorship and Annexe. (3/1995, 25 January) London: UKCC.

Report of the Committee on Nursing (1972) Chairman, Professor Asa Briggs. Cmnd 5115. London: HMSO.

Richardson G, Maynard A (1995) Fewer Doctors? More Nurses? A Review of the Knowledge Base of Doctor–Nurse Substitution. Discussion Paper 135. York: University of York, Centre for Health Economics, York Health Economics Consortium, NHS Centre for Reviews and Dissemination.

Riddell MS (1914) Lectures to Nurses. London: The Scientific Press Limited. (2nd edn, 1925; 3rd edn, 1928; 4th edn, 1931; 5th edn, 1933; 6th edn, 1936)

Riddell MS (1931) A First Year Nursing Manual. London: The Scientific Press, Faber and Faber Limited. (2nd edn, 1934; 3rd edn, 1936; 4th edn, 1937; 5th edn, 1939)

Ridge KW, Jenkins DB, Noyce PR, Barber ND (1995) Medication errors during hospital drug rounds. Quality in Health Care 4: 240–43.

Rivett G (1998) From Cradle to Grave: Fifty Years of the NHS. London: King's Fund.

Robinson J (1993) Three Years on: Experiences of a Project 2000 Demonstration District. Suffolk and Great Yarmouth College of Nursing and Midwifery with Suffolk College.

Robinson D, Buchan J, Hayday S (1999) On the Agenda: Changing Nurses' Careers in 1999. Brighton: University of Sussex, Institute of Employment Studies.

Robinson J, Leamon J (1999) A Documentary Analysis of Educational Programmes Leading to the Award of Degree in Nursing at Pre and Post-registration Level. London: ENB.

Robinson S, Inyang V (1999) The nurse practitioner in emergency medicine – valuable but undefined. The Lancet 354: 1319–20.

Rodgers S (1998) Treated or mistreated? The Guardian Society p. 3, August 26.

Rowden R (1984a) Doctors can work with the nursing process, a reply to Professor Mitchell. British Medical Journal 288: 219–21.

Rowden R (1984b) Doctors can work with the nursing process, a reply to Professor Mitchell. Nursing Times 80(19): 32–34.

Royal College of Physicians (2000) Hospital Doctors Under Pressure: New Roles for the Health Care Workforce. London: Royal College of Physicians. April.

Sakra M, Angus J, Perrin J, Nixon G, Nicholl J, Wardrope J (1999) Care of minor injuries by emergency nurse practitioners or junior doctors, a randomised controlled trial. The Lancet 354: 1321–26.

Salter B, Snee N (1997) Power dressing. Health Service Journal, 13 February: 30–31.

Salvage J (1985) The Politics of Nursing. London: Heinemann.

Salvage J (1988) Thumbs up from government for reform of nurse training. British Medical Journal 296: 1553.

Salvage J, Smith R (2000a) Who wears the trousers? Nursing Times 96(15): 24.

Salvage J, Smith R (2000b) Doctors and nurses: doing it differently. British Medical Journal 320: 1019–20.

Scales M (1952) Handbook for Ward Sisters. London: Baillière, Tindall and Cox. (2nd edn, 1958)

Scarth A (1997) Sick to death of nursing. The Guardian (Education Supplement, Higher Education, On Campus), 8 April: iv.

Scholes J, Endacott R, Chellel A (1999) Diversity and Complexity: A Documentary Analysis of Critical Care Nursing Education. Researching Professional Education Research, Report Series No. 13. London: ENB.

SCAA (1997) Literacy and numeracy in the workplace. London: School Curriculum and Assessment Authority.

Scott H (1997) Healthcare assistants: the substitute nurse (editorial). British Journal of Nursing 6(19): 1092, October 23.

Sears WG (1953), Medicine for Nurses. London: Edward Arnold. (2nd edn, 1937; 3rd edn, 1939; 4th edn, 1945; 5th edn, 1949; 6th edn, 1954; 7th edn, 1957; 8th edn, 1960; 9th edn, 1963; with Winwood RS, 10th edn, 1966; 11th edn, 1970; 12th edn, 1975; 13th edn, 1979)

Seccombe I, Smith G (1997) Taking Part: Registered Nurses and the Labour Market in 1997. The Institute for Employment Studies, Report 338. Brighton: University of Sussex.

Seccombe I, Smith G (1998) Changing Times: A Survey of Registered Nurses in 1998. The Institute for Employment Studies, Report 351. Brighton: University of Sussex.

Secretary of State for Health (2000a) The NHS Plan: A Plan for Investment, A Plan for Reform. Cm 4818-I. London: Department of Health.

Secretary of State for Health (2000b) The NHS Plan: The Government's Response to the Royal Commission on Long Term Care. Cm 4818-II. London: Department of Health.

Serious Hazards of Transfusion (2000) Annual Report 1998–1999. Manchester: Manchester Blood Centre. April.

Sewell B (1999) Bring on the bedpan brigade. Evening Standard, 12 January: 15.

Sharp L (1997) Too many cowboys but not enough Indians. Nursing Times (Letters) 93(20): 20.

Shelley H (1997) It's all academic. Nursing Times 93(2): 49.

Sherrington K (1997) First class nursing without degrees. Nursing Standard 12(8):18.

Singh A (1970) The student nurse on experimental courses – I: Attitudes towards nursing as a career. International Journal of Nursing Studies 7: 201–24.

Singh A (1971a) The student nurse on experimental courses – II: Personality patterns. International Journal of Nursing Studies 8: 189–205.

Singh A (1971b) The student nurse on experimental courses – III: Basic values. International Journal of Nursing Studies 8: 207–18.

Singh A, MacGuire J (1971) Occupational values and stereotypes in a group of trained nurses. Nursing Times (Occasional Papers) 67(42): 165–68.

Skyte S (1998) Reviewing the situation. Nursing Standard 12(50): 52–53.

Skyte S (1999) Help, we need somebody. Nursing Standard 14(4): 69.

Smith EM (1929) Notes on Practical Nursing. London: Faber and Gwyer Ltd.

Smith P (1992) The Emotional Labour of Nursing. Basingstoke: Macmillan.

Smith P, Masterson A, Lloyd Smith S (1999) Health promotion versus disease and care, failure to establish "blissful clarity" in British nurse education and practice. Social Science and Medicine 48: 227–39.

Stannard C (1978) Old folks and dirty work, the social conditions for patient abuse in a nursing home. In Dingwall R, McIntosh J, (Eds) Readings in the Sociology of Nursing. Edinburgh: Churchill Livingstone. pp 164–80.

Statutory Instruments (1983) Nurses, Midwives and Health Visitors Rules Approval order 1983, No 873. London: HMSO.

Statutory Instruments (1989) Nurses, Midwives and Health Visitors: The Nurses, Midwives and Health Visitors (Registered Fever Nurses Amendment Rules and Training Amendment Rules) Approval Order 1989, No1456. London: HMSO.

Stewart I, Cuff HE (1899) Practical Nursing. Edinburgh and London: William Blackwood and Sons. (2nd edn, 1903; new edn, 1904; 3rd edn, 1910; 4th edn, 1913)

Stokes HC, Thompson DR, Seers K (1998) The implementation of multiprofessional guidelines for cardiac rehabilitation, a pilot study. Coronary Health Care 2: 60–71.

Stott E (1999) 'We get plenty of practice . . .' Nursing Times (Letters) 95(42): 21.

Stott F (1998) Nursing by the book. Sunday Telegraph (Letters to the Editor), 22 February: 34.

Stott F (1999) Nursing shortage. The Times (Letters to the Editor), 13 January: 19.

Strong S (1997) Unconditional Love? London: The Mental Health Foundation.

The Times (1995) Complaints double over 'uncaring' NHS. The Times, 14 July: 8

The Times (1997) Student nurse shortage 'is threat to NHS'. The Times, 22 November: 4.

Thomas LH, MacMillan J, McColl E, Priest J, Hale C, Bond S (1995) Obtaining patients' views of nursing care to inform the development of a patient satisfaction scale. International Journal for Quality in Health Care 7(2): 153–63.

Thornley C (1997a) The Invisible Workers: An Investigation into the Pay and Employment of Health Care Assistants in the NHS. London: Unison Health Care.

Thornley C (1997b) Phantoms of the hospital. Nursing Times 93(42): 18.

Thornley C (1998a) Neglected Nurses, Hidden Work: An Investigation into the Pay and Employment of Nursing Auxiliaries and Assistants in the NHS. London: Unison Health Care.

Thornley C (1998b) Ignored and unrewarded. Nursing Times 94(41): 15.

Thornley C (1999) Out of Sight, Out of Mind. London: Unison Health Care.

Titmuss RM (1970) The Gift Relationship: From Human Blood to Social Relationship. London: George Allen and Unwin.

Todd CJ, Freeman CJ, Camilleri-Ferrante C, Palmer CR, Hyder A, Laxton CE, Parker MJ, Payne BV, Rushton N (1995) Differences in mortality after fracture of hip, the East Anglian audit. British Medical Journal 310: 904–8.

Tompsett KR (1998) Training and pay behind haemorrhage of NHS staff. The Times (Letters to the Editor), 11 August: 17.

Toohey M (1953) Medicine for Nurses. Edinburgh: E and S Livingstone. (2nd edn, 1955; 3rd edn, 1957; 4th edn, 1959; 5th edn, 1960; 6th edn, 1963; 7th edn, 1965; 8th edn, 1967; 9th edn, 1969; 10th edn, 1971; 11th edn, 1975; 12th edn, 1978; 13th edn, 1981; 14th edn, 1986)

Tooley J, Darby D (1998) Educational Research – A Critique: A Survey of Published Educational Research. London: Office for Standards in Education.

Traynor M (1999) Managerialism and Nursing. London: Routledge.

Traynor M, Rafferty AM (1998) Nursing Research and the Higher Education Context: A Second Working Paper. London: Centre for Policy in Nursing Research. March.

Turner T, Dickson N (1988) Project 2000: a new dawn for nursing? Nursing Times 84(22): 12–13.

UKCC (1984) Code of Professional Conduct. 2nd edn. London: UKCC.

UKCC (1986a) Project 2000: A New Preparation for Practice. London: UKCC.

UKCC (1986b) Project 2000: The Project and the Professions: Results of the UKCC Consultation on Project 2000. Project Paper 7, November. London: UKCC.

UKCC (1987a) Project 2000: Counting the Cost: Is Project 2000 a Practical Proposition? Project Paper 8, February. London: UKCC.

UKCC (1987b) Project 2000: The Final Proposals. February. London: UKCC.

UKCC (1988) Proposed Rules for the Standard, Kind and Content of Future Pre-registration Nursing Education. London: UKCC.

UKCC (1989a) Exercising Accountability. London: UKCC.

UKCC (1989b) UKCC Requirements for the Content of Project 2000 Programmes PS and D/89/04 (B). London: UKCC.

UKCC (1990) The Report of the Post-registration education and Practice Project. London: UKCC.

UKCC (1992a) Code of Professional Conduct, 3rd edn. London: UKCC.

UKCC (1992b) The Scope of Professional Practice. London: UKCC.

UKCC (1994a) The Future of Professional Practice – The Council's Standards for Education and Practice following Registration. London: UKCC.

UKCC (1994b) PREP – Government supports UKCC proposals. Register 14: 4–5. Spring.

UKCC (1995) PREP and you – your questions answered. Register 16: 4–5. Winter.

UKCC (1996a) Guidelines for Professional Practice. London: UKCC.

UKCC (1996b) PREP and profiling. Register17: 8–9. Summer.

UKCC (1996c) Issues Arising from Professional Complaints. London: UKCC.

UKCC (1997a) "UKCC – can I help you?" Seeking professional advice. Register 20: 8. Summer.

UKCC (1997b) The Future of Professional Regulation: Submission of the UKCC to the Government's Review of the Nurses, Midwives and Health Visitors Act (1997). London: UKCC. December.

UKCC (1998a) A Higher Level of Practice: Consultation Document. London: UKCC.

UKCC (1998b) UKCC Education Commission: Terms of Reference, 18 March.

UKCC (1998c) Abuse of patients and inappropriate relationships between patients and practitioners. Register 24: 9. Summer.

UKCC (1999a) Fitness for Practice: The UKCC Commission for Nursing and Midwifery Education. Chair, Sir Leonard Peach London: UKCC.

UKCC (1999b) A Higher Level of Practice. London: UKCC. April.

UKCC (1999c) Practitioner-Client Relationships and the Prevention of Abuse. London: UKCC. September.

UKCC (1999d) Statistical Analysis of the UKCC's Professional Register, 1 April 1998 to 31 March 1999. London: UKCC. November.

UKCC (1999e) The future of professional regulation. Register 29: 5. Autumn.

UKCC (2000a) The Scope of Professional Practice – A Study of its Implementation. London: UKCC. January.

UKCC (2000b) Requirements for Pre-Registration Nursing Programmes. London: UKCC. May.

UKCC Commission for Nursing and Midwifery Education (1998) UKCC Education Commission Attitudinal Survey. BMRB International and UKCC. September.

UKCC, Educational Policy Advisory Committee (1985a) Project 2000: Introducing Project 2000. Project Paper 1, September. London: UKCC.

UKCC, Educational Policy Advisory Committee (1985b) Project 2000: The Learner: Student Status Revisited. Project Paper 2, September. London: UKCC.

UKCC, Educational Policy Advisory Committee (1985c) Project 2000: One-Two-Three How Many Levels of Nurse Should There Be? Project Paper 3, September. London, UKCC.

UKCC, Educational Policy Advisory Committee (1985d) Project 2000: The Enrolled Nurse: Looking Back and Looking Forward. Project Paper 4, September. London: UKCC.

UKCC, Educational Policy Advisory Committee (1985e) Project 2000: Redrawing The Boundaries. Project Paper 5, November. London: UKCC.

UKCC, Educational Policy Advisory Committee (1985f) Project 2000: Facing the Future. Project Paper 6, November. London: UKCC.

UKCC News Online (2000a) Ensuring effective public protection. http://www.ukcc.org.uk/news2.htm

UKCC News Online (2000b) Professional Conduct annual report 1999–2000. http://www.ukcc.org.uk/news2.htm

Unison Health Care (1997) Condition Critical: The Crisis in Nursing Pay, Unison's evidence to the Nurses, Midwives and Health Visitors Pay Review Body 1998. London: Unison.

University of Exeter (1996) Mathematical Needs of Young Employees in Business, Industry and the Public Services: Final Report for SCAA. University of Exeter, Centre for Innovation in Mathematics Teaching, March.

USA Today (19999) Nurses and quality of care (Part I) Nurse-staffing laws inadequate salve for hospitals' wounds. Our view. Patients lack of information, choice, which demand deeper reforms. USA Today, 18 October: 18A.

Vivian M (1920) Lectures to Nurses in Training. London: The Scientific Press.

Vousden M (1998) Nursing a grievance. Nursing Times 94(26): 18–19.

Voysey MHA (1905) Nursing: Hints to Probationers on Practical Work. London: The Scientific Press. (Revised 1911)

Wake R (1998) The Nightingale Training School 1860–1996. London: Haggerston Press.

Wal L (1999) Is Project 2000 ready for 2000? Nursing Times 95(39): 17.

Wallace H, Mulcahy L (1999) Cause for Complaint: An Evaluation of the Effectiveness of the NHS Complaints Procedure. Public Law Project, Birkbeck College, University of London.

Walsh M, Ford P (1989) Nursing Rituals: Research and Rational Actions. Oxford: Butterworth-Heinemann Ltd.

Warner M, Longley M, Gould E, Picek A (1998) Healthcare Futures 2010: Commissioned by the UKCC Education Commission. Pontypridd: University of Glamorgan, Welsh Institute for Health and Social Care. December.

Warnock M (1985) Teacher teach thyself. The 1985 Richard Dimbleby Lecture. The Listener, 28 March: 10–14.

Warnock M (1988) A Common Policy for Education. Oxford: Oxford University Press.

Warren J, Harris M (1998) Extinguishing the lamp: the crisis in nursing. In Digby A, (Ed) Come Back Miss Nightingale. London: Social Affairs Unit. pp 1–35.

Waterlow J (1999) Sacrificial lambs. Nursing Times 95(39): 30–31.

Watson H, Harris B (1999) Supporting Students in Practice Placements in Scotland. Glasgow: Glasgow Caledonian University, Department of Nursing and Community Health.

Watt N (1998) New rota system could solve nursing crisis. The Times, 23 February: 2.

Wharrad HJ, Allcock N, Chapple M (1994) A survey of the teaching and learning of biological sciences on undergraduate nursing courses. Nurse Education Today 14: 436–42.

While A (1994) Competence versus performance, which is more important? Journal of Advanced Nursing 20: 525–31.

While A (1996) Strengths in diversity, interview by Potrykus C. Nursing Standard 10(15): 51.

While A, Roberts J, Fitzpatrick J (1995) A Comparative Study of Outcomes of Pre-Registration Nurse Education Programmes. London: ENB.

White E, Riley E, Davies S, Twinn S (1993) A Detailed Study of the Relationships between Teaching, Support, Supervision and Role Modelling in Clinical Areas, within the Context of Project 2000 Courses. London: ENB.

White BJ (1998) A nurse's experience. In Kilner JF, Orr RD, Shelly JA, (Eds) The Changing Face of Health Care. Grand Rapids: Wm B Eerdmans. pp 17–32.

Wilkinson R (1996) Nurses, concerns about IV therapy and devices. Nursing Standard 10(35): 35–37.

Willcock K (1997) The Tip of the Iceberg: A Survey of Complaints Registered by Community Health Councils Concerning the Care of Older People in NHS Hospitals. London: Help the Aged. October.

Williams C, Soothill K, Barry J (1992) Nursing wastage from the nurses' perspective. In Soothill K, Henry C, Kendrick K (Eds) Themes and Perspectives in Nursing. London: Chapman and Hall. pp 214–30.

Williams S, Michie S, Pattani S (1998) Improving the Health of the NHS Workforce. Nuffield Trust Report. London: The Nuffield Trust.

Williams K (1978) Ideologies of nursing, their meanings and implications. In Dingwall R, McIntosh J (Eds) Readings in the Sociology of Nursing. Edinburgh: Churchill Livingstone. pp 36–44.

Williams L (1999) Prepared to pull my weight. Nursing Times (Letters) 95(42): 20–21.

Williams M (1999) Auditing the PREP standards for ensuring fitness to practise. Nursing Times 95(49): 55–56.

Williams R, Fisher A (1877) Hints for Hospital Nurses. Edinburgh: MacLachlan and Stewart. London: Simpkin, Marshall and Co. Dublin: Fannin and Co.

Williamson J (1998) Nursing grudges. Sunday Telegraph (Letters to the Editor), 1 March: 32.

Wilson-Barnett J (1986a) Professional issues. Nursing Times 82(42): 53–55.

Wilson-Barnett J (1986b) Ethical dilemmas in nursing. Journal of Medical Ethics 12: 123–26, 135.

Winson SKG (1995) Demographic differences between degree and diploma student nurses. Nursing Standard 9(23): 35–38.

Wood CJ (undated, c.1887) A Handbook of Nursing for the Home and the Hospital. 8th edn. London: Cassell and Co.

Wright S (1998) An eye to the future. Nursing Standard 12(48): 20–22.

Wright S, Gough P, Poulton B (1998) Imagine the Future: The Full Report of the RCN Futures Project. London: RCN.

Wyatt JF (1978) Sociological perspectives on socialization into a profession: a study of student nurses and their definition of learning. British Journal of Educational Studies, vol. XXVI(3): 263–76.

Yorston, J (1997) More nurses need academic abilities. Nursing Standard 12(11): 11.

Index

1919 Nurses' Registration Act 1, 2
1979 Nurses, Midwives and Health
Visitors Act 14, 15, 18, 24, 37, 70, 73, 151, 154, 161, 171, 183, 185
1983 Rules Approval order, statutory instrument 24, 25, 49
1989 Rules Approval order, statutory instrument 36, 37, 49
1991–1992 Nurses, Midwives and Health Visitors Bill 151–61
1997 Review of the Nurses, Midwives and Health Visitors Act 171, 183
1999 Health Bill 171
1999 Health Act 173

A Higher Level of Practice 98, 99
A Structure for Nursing 18, 19, 20, 21
Abel-Smith B 12
Addenbrooke's Hospital 5
Addington, Lord 167
Age Concern 122, 137
Aiken LH, Smith HL, Lake ET 119
Alderman C 105
Allen C 58
Allman DJ 110
Amos, Baroness 167
Appleyard W J 20, 42
apprenticeship xi, xii, 1–18, 23, 25, 38, 39, 40, 43, 45, 71, 83, 84, 92, 93, 102, 107, 110, 111, 114, 137, 166, 175, 179, 183, 185–7
Ashdown AM 6
Ashworth PD, Gerrish K, Hargreaves J, McManus M 178
Association of Community Health Councils 122, 123

Atkinson E 110
Auckland, Lord 153
Audit Commission 95, 97

Baldwin N 136
Barrett J 91
Bartlett HP, Simonte V, Westcott E, Taylor HR 68
Bedford H, Phillips T, Robinson J, Schostak J 56, 57
Bedford Fenwick E 22
Bendall E 13
Berners, Baroness 172
Berry M 134
Bevan N 170
Binnie A, Titchen A 147
Birmingham General Hospital 8
Blegen MA, Goode CJ, Reed L 120
Bliss M 102, 103, 149
Bond S, Thomas LH 126
Booth B 107
Bottomley V 154–62, 170–4
Boyle S
Bradley P 133
Bradshaw A vii, x, 1, 11, 14, 47, 50
Bradshaw R 140
Bree-Williams FJ, Waterman H 66
Bridgeman, Viscount 181
Briggs, Lord (Asa) 13, 14, 16
Bright M 122, 128
Brignall J 107, 108
Brindle D 82, 121
British Journal of Nursing 90, 91
British Medical Journal 18, 21, 41,43, 85, 94, 97, 178
Brookes Y, Bristoll C, Young B 109

Brown DF 110
Bryceworth D 6
Buchan J 115
Buchan J, Seccombe I, Smith G 116
Bullivant D 87
Butterworth T 69

Caines E 94, 118
Campbell R 134, 135, 136
Cantrill P 134, 135
Carers' National Association 123, 124
Carlisle D 154
Carpenter M 142, 143
Carr-Hill R, Dixon P, Gibbs I, et al 90, 91, 121
Carter, Lord 153
Cartwright A 125
Casey N, Smith R 94, 105
Castledine G 21, 56
Central Committee for Hospital Medical Services 18, 19, 20, 41
Chapman P 92, 179
Charnley E 65
Christie R 112
Clark J 79, 91, 175
Clarke K 15, 89
Clarke M 10
clinical governance 164, 170
Clinton, HR 119
Cochrane DA, Conroy M 93, 99
Cochrane DA, Conroy M, Crilly T and Rogers J 99, 100, 101
Cochrane M 7
Cohen G 20
Commission for Health Improvement 170, 173
Community Health Council 139
Council of Deans and Heads 91
Council for National Academic Awards (CNAA) 152
Cox C 152, 153, 181
Cox C, Lewin D, Hewins S, Bowman K 23, 24, 25
Croft J 5, 6
Cullum N, Dickson R, Eastwood A 67
Cumberlege J 96, 152, 153, 154, 164, 165

Cundy J M 20, 42
Cutting KF 66

Daily Mail vii, 110
Daily Express 110
Daily Telegraph 137, 181
Dannatt A 6, 8
Darley M 111
Davies C 33, 35, 40, 41, 43, 44, 48, 178, 179
Davies C, Beach A 179
Davies L 112
Davis F 146
Davis M 107
Davison G 109
Day H, James P 109
De Witt R 52
Dean M 88
Deegan M 64, 65
Delamothe T 43
De Moro RA 120
Denham J 117, 175
Devlin B 42
Department of Education 154
Department of Health 62, 86, 98, 134, 174, 175, 177, 178, 182
Dewar J 41
Dickson N 42, 45
'Dignity on the Ward' campaign 137
Dingwall R, McIntosh J 146
Dingwall R, Rafferty AM, Webster C 32
Dobson F 116, 135, 136, 161, 169, 170, 172, 175, 176
Domville EJ 5
Dorrell S 161
Dowling S, Barrett S, West R 97
Doyal L, Dowling S, Cameron A 97
Drown J 91
Duffy Y 109
Dunn M 116
Dunwoody G 155
Dutton A 14, 41
Dyson R 110, 111

Earnshaw C 109
Edinburgh Royal Infirmary 4
Education Purchasing Consortia 93

Elder J 173
Elkan R, Hillman R, Robinson J 57, 58
Emerton A vii, 30, 43, 44, 89, 166, 167,
    171, 172, 181
Emmet DM 10
English National Board for Nursing,
    Midwifery and Health Visiting
    (ENB) viii, xii, 13, 18, 22, 26, 27,
    30, 31, 32, 38, 47–57, 64, 73, 77,
    78, 80, 116, 156, 174, 182
ENB syllabus and regulations 22, 26, 27,
    30, 49–57, 60, 174
English T 94
Eraut M, Alderton J, Boylan A, Wraight A
    59

Fabricius J 148, 149
Fawkes BN 13
Fearon M 71
Felix C 109
Ferriman A 85
Fever Hospital, Newcastle-upon-Tyne 4
Finlayson LR, Nazroo JY 105, 128
Fisher A 4, 8, 9
Fisher E 5
Fisher P 102
Fitzpatrick R 128
Flatt S 108
Fleming J 33, 40
Foskett NH, Hemsley-Brown JV 86, 87,
    105, 167
Fox EM 9
Francis B, Peelo M, Soothill K 105
Freidson E 11,12
Fyfe M 158, 159, 160, 161

Gaba M 102
Gabbittass G 110
General Medical Council (GMC) 94, 155,
    156
General Nursing Council (GNC) 1, 2, 3,
    12, 23, 70, 71
GNC syllabus 1, 2, 3, 66, 70, 143
George S 111
gender and nursing 43,44, 86, 87, 101,
    105, 142, 143, 178, 183, 185–7
Gerrish K, McManus M, Ashworth P 60
Ghazi F, Henshaw L 66

Gibberd B 42
Gillespie A, Curzio J, 67
Gillon R 101, 102
Girvin J 107
Glen J 109
Gloucestershire Community Health
    Council 128
Godfrey K 67
Goldhill DR, Worthington LM, Mulcahy
    AJ, Tarling MM 97
Goodwin L, Bosanquet N 32
Gott M 23
Gough P 99
Gould M 96
Gould D, Chamberlain A 66
graduate status 23, 82, 91, 92
Graham, Lord 167
Gration HM 7
Gration HM, Holland DL 7
Greenwood RK 20
Grüneberg A 42
Guardian 82, 108, 117, 121, 128, 171
Gulland A, O'Dowd A 117
Guy's Hospital 8

Hadley W 6
Hallam J 144
Handy C 48
Harding-Price D 109
Harper M 111
Harris M 118
Harvey LP 20, 42
Hay R 102
Hayman, Baroness 171
Heal S 155, 157, 160
Health Advisory Service 129, 130
health care assistant/nursing auxiliary/
    support worker xiii, 20, 36, 44, 45,
    63, 64, 76–8, 88, 89, 90, 91, 92, 95,
    99, 100–3, 108, 112, 118, 120, 135,
    137, 139, 140, 147, 153, 168, 173,
    178, 183
Health Manpower Management 110
Health Service Commissioner
    (Ombudsman) 121, 122, 130, 131,
    136, 138, 139, 164, 181
Hector W 170
Hek G 61

Help the Aged 137, 142
Henwood M 123, 124
Hewison J 92
Hewison J, Millar B, Dowswell T 93
Higgins B, Hurst K, Wistow G 128
Hinchliffe D 156, 157, 158, 159
Hinde J 65
Hobbs R, Murray ET 97
Hooper J 55
Hooper, Baroness 153, 154
Hopkins R 20
Horton R 102
Hospital for Sick Children, Great
    Ormond Street 5
Houghton M 10
House of Commons 15, 90, 122, 130–6,
    139, 151, 154–61, 169, 170–75,
    180, 181, 183
House of Lords vii, x, xi, 9, 14, 15, 16,
    103, 137, 151–4, 162–9, 171, 172,
    181, 183
Howe, Earl vii, 167, 168
Huehns T 126
Humphry L 5
Hunt, Lord vii, 165, 166, 181
Hutt R, Connor H, Hirsh W 28, 34
Hutton J 117

Incomes Data Services 115, 116, 117
Independent 117
Institute of Employment Studies 94

Jacka K, Lewin D 38, 39
James P, Day H 109
Jay M vii, 115, 168, 169
Jeffries H 72
Jenkins S 109
Jenkinson T 112
JM Consulting 73–8, 98, 141, 161, 171
Johnson M 132, 133
Joint Consultants Committee 21
Jones L, Leneman L, Maclean U 126
Jordan S, Potter N 67
Jowett S, Walton I, Payne S 57, 58
Judge H 30, 32, 33, 40

Katz FE 146, 147
Keen, A 172

Kenward D 20
Kershaw B 166
Kershaw L 137
King E 110
King's College, London 111
King's Fund 182
Kitson A 119
Kratz C 35

Lancet Report 166
Langlands A 135, 136
Lask S, Smith P, Masterson A 59
Latter S, Yerrell P, Rycroft-Malone J,
    Shaw D 67
Lawson N 118
Lavin M 72
Lees F 4, 8
Le Fanu J 102
Le Grand J 149
Lelean SR 10
Lewis EB 20
Lewis PG 6
Lilley R 118
Lipley N 79
London Hospital 5, 6
Longhurst RH 67
Lückes E 5
Luker KA, Carlisle C, Riley E, Stilwell J,
    Davies C, Wilson R 61–5, 68
Luker KA, Hogg C, Austin L, Ferguson B,
    Smith K 95,96

MacGuire J 14, 29, 145
Mackay L 41, 43, 104
MacKenzie H 103, 181
Macleod Clark J, Maben J, Jones K 57, 59
magnet hospitals 119
Making a Difference 174, 175
Marrin M 118
Marsh DC Willcocks AJ 14
Masham, Baroness vii, 165, 181
matron x, 2, 3, 5, 6, 7, 9, 11, 20, 102,
    165, 182, 189
May N, Veitch L, McIntosh JB, Alexander
    MF 61
May P 102
Maynard A 99, 184
McColl, Lord x

McFarlane J vii, 21–3, 103, 151–3, 166, 171, 172, 181
McManus IC, Richards P, Winder BC, Sproston KA 65, 81, 96
McTaggart F 132
Meadows S, Levenson R, Baeza J 182
Medical Devices Agency 67
Mencap 122, 123
Menzies IEP (later Menzies-Lyth) 12, 41, 147, 148
Mercator 104
Meredith P 125, 126
Meredith P, Wood C 124
Meston, Lord 153
Middlesex Hospital 5
Milburn A 116, 177, 178, 179
Mills M 110
Mitchell J R A 21, 22
Moore J 43–5, 89, 151, 153
Moores B 34
Moores Y 64, 65, 161
Morgan O 120
Morgan R 131–4, 136
Moroney J 6
Morris A 109
Morris B (Lord) vii, viii, ix, x, 162–4, 167, 181
Morton-Williams J, Berthoud R 29
Mullally S 176, 177
Munro R 111
Murray T 109

National Audit Office 38, 56, 180
National Boards 73, 76–8, 151, 153, 156–61, 171, 182, 183, 189
National Committee of Inquiry into Higher Education (Chairman: Sir Ron Dearing) 76
National Consumer Council 173
National Institute for Clinical Excellence 136, 170
National Vocational Qualifications 45, 77, 89, 90
Neary M 65, 66
Nessling RC 43, 103, 104
New End Hospital, Hampstead 5
The New NHS 91, 95, 161, 162
The NHS Plan 181

Newton G 92
NHS Direct 164, 168, 184
NHS Executive 90, 92, 97, 134, 135, 139, 142, 161, 162, 170, 171, 175, 176, 178, 179, 180
Nicklin P, Kenworthy N 55, 56
Nightingale School 5
Nightingale F vii, ix, 10, 11, 22, 109, 129, 143
Norman S 72, 73
North American nursing 21, 35, 95, 119, 120, 146, 150, 175
North Tees General Hospital 42
Nuffield Trust 116
Nurses' (Nurse's) Chart/ Record of Practical Instruction and Experience 2,3, 64, 70, 71
Nurses' Council 173, 177
Nursing and Midwifery Council 182
Nurses, Midwives and Health Visitors Pay Review Body 88, 182
nursing development units 98
nurse consultants 97
nurse (health care) practitioner 94, 96, 97, 99–102, 152, 155, 165, 168
nurse prescribing 51, 95, 96, 152, 155, 164, 178
nursing process 21, 22
Nursing Standard 70, 72, 73, 79, 82, 94, 97, 98, 99, 100, 104, 108, 109, 115–18, 140, 141, 175–7, 182
Nursing Times 11, 13, 21, 42, 45, 70, 72, 73, 78, 82, 88, 91, 92, 95, 102, 103, 107, 111, 112, 115–7, 121, 122, 130, 141, 144, 154, 171, 176–8, 182
nursing values/ethos of care viii, ix, xi, xii, xiii, 4, 5, 16, 36, 49, 48, 68, 74, 76, 83, 85–7, 91, 101–14, 118–24, 129, 131–49, 163, 166, 167, 169, 170, 172, 178, 183–7

O'Dowd A 67
Ogden J 154
Oxford Mail 116
Oxford MN 7
Oxford Times 116

Parry-Jones WLI 14
Parsons T 10
Patient's Charter 157, 169
Peach L 79, 80, 176
Pearce EC 5, 7, 10, 12, 119, 142
Peelo M, Francis B, Soothill K 105
Pembrey S. 18–20
Pendry T 156–8, 161
Phillips M 118
Phillips T, Schostak J, Bedford H, Leamon J 60, 61
Phillips T, Schostak J, Tyler J, Allen L 68
Poulton K 34
Practitioner-Client Relationships and the Prevention of Abuse 141
PREP 68, 69, 70, 73, 102, 160
Preston and County of Lancaster Royal Infirmary and Fever Hospital 6
Price Waterhouse 103
Prince of Wales Hospital, Tottenham 9
'professionhood'/professionalization viii, 11, 85, 101, 105, 179, 188, 190
Project 2000 ix, xi, xii, 27, 31, 33–8, 41–5, 47, 56–67, 75, 79, 80, 82, 83, 85, 103, 106, 107, 110–12, 114, 119, 120, 134, 150–154, 157–160, 163, 164, 166, 172, 181, 182, 185, 189, 191
Psychoanalytic Psychotherapy 148
Purdy R 110

Qualpacs 121
Quality Assurance Agency 76, 77, 174
Queen's speech xi

Ralph C 154
Raven K 118, 119
recruitment, retention, nurse shortages xiii, 34, 38, 42, 80, 88, 90, 94, 100, 110, 112–8, 142–4, 146, 149, 150, 154, 162–9, 182, 183, 188, 189
Redfern S, Norman I, Murrells T, Christian S, Gilmore A, Normand C, Stevens W Langham S 98
Report of the Committee on Nurse Education, 1964 (Chairman: Sir Robert Platt) 12
Report of the Committee on Nursing, 1972 (Chairman: Asa Briggs) viii, ix, xi,13, 14, 16, 18, 29, 32, 47, 144
Report of the Committee on Senior Nursing Staff, 1966 (Chairman: Brian Salmon) 32
revisionist history 142–4
Richardson G, Maynard A 94, 95
Riddell MS 7
Ridge KW, Jenkins DB, Noyce PR, Barber ND 66
Rivett G 102, 103, 118, 120, 129, 149, 169, 175
Robinson J 57, 58
Robinson D, Buchan J, Hayday S 117
Robinson J, Leamon J 68, 174
Robinson S, Inyang V 96
Robson, Baroness 154
Rodgers S 136
Ross APJ 20
Rowden R 21, 22
Royal College of Nursing (RCN) xii, 12, 18–21, 27, 28, 29, 30, 31, 44, 47, 73, 76, 77, 88, 91, 92, 93, 99, 105–7, 109, 110, 115, 116, 117, 129, 144, 162, 164, 165, 167, 175, 178, 180, 182
RCN Commission on Nursing Education (Chairman: Harry Judge) viiii, 27, 28, 29, 20, 27–34, 38, 40
Royal College of Physicians 178
Royal College of Surgeons 124, 125
Royal Commission on long-term care 180
Royal Devon and Exeter Hospital 5
Royal Infirmary, Manchester 6
Rye D 18, 19, 21

Sakra M, Angus J, Perrin J, Nixon G, Nicholl J, Wardrope J 96
Salop Infirmary 6
Salter B, Snee N 99
Salvage J 45, 143
Salvage J, Smith R 178
Scales M 8, 9
Scarth A 108
Social and Community Planning Research (SCPR) 29
Scholes J, Endacott R, Chellel A 97

School Curriculum and Assessment
  Authority (SCAA) 61
The Scotsman 110, 111
Scott H 90
Sears WG 6
Seccombe I, Smith G 94, 115
Serious Hazards of Transfusion (SHOT)
  180
Sewell B 118
Shaping the Future 91
Sharp L 108
Shelley H 107
Shephard G 42, 43
Sherrington K 108, 109
Sims R 155, 159
Singh A 14
Singh A, MacGuire J 14
Singleton C 108
Skyte S 79, 99
Smith A 52
Smith EM 7
Smith, Lord 15, 16, 151
Smith P 143, 145
Smith P, Masterson A, Lloyd Smith S 67,
  68, 81
Southampton Infirmary 6
specialist nursing 50, 51, 94–9, 115, 152,
  164
Stannard C 146
St Bartholomew's Hospital 102
St Mary's Hospital 4
St Thomas's Hospital xi, 2, 4, 6
Sterling N 42
Stewart I, Cuff HE 6
Stoddart, Lord 169
Stokes HC, Thompson DR, Seers K 96
Stott E 112
Stott F 110, 118
Strategy for Nursing 161
Strong S 121

The Times 110, 115, 116, 121
Times Higher Education Supplement 65
Thomas LH, MacMillan J, McColl E, Priest
  J, Hale C, Bond S 126, 127, 128
Thornley C 88, 89, 90, 95
Titmuss RM 149

Todd CJ, Freeman CJ, Camilleri-Ferrante
  C, Palmer CR, Hyder A, Laxton CE,
  Parker MJ, Payne BV, Rushton, N 66
Tompsett KR 110
Toohey M 6
Tooley J, Darby D 107
Towards Standards 18–21
Traynor M 105
Traynor M, Rafferty AM 91
Turner T, Dickson N 45
Universities and Colleges Admissions
  Service (UCAS) 116
United Kingdom Central Council for
  Nursing, Midwifery and Health
  Visiting (UKCC) viii, xi, xii, 15, 18,
  27, 31, 33–5, 36–8, 40, 41–5, 47,
  50, 53, 56, 57, 62, 64, 68, 69, 70,
  72–76, 78–82, 84, 89, 91, 93, 98,
  99, 114, 117, 120, 129, 130, 140,
  141, 142, 151–61, 166–9, 171, 173,
  178, 179, 180, 182, 183, 189
UKCC Commission on Nursing and
  Midwifery Education (Chairman:
  Sir Leonard Peach) 78–82, 98, 175,
  176
UKCC codes of conduct 62
UKCC professional conduct 72–4, 76,
  140, 141, 142, 152
Unison 88, 89, 90, 92, 116, 179
University of Exeter 161
University of Manchester 10, 22
Uprichard M 91
USA Today 120

Victoria Hospital, Folkstone 6
Vivian M 7
vocation and nursing viii, x, xii, xiii, 5,
  10, 11, 12, 16, 41, 43, 85, 101,
  104, 105, 108, 110, 112, 118,
  142–7, 149, 163, 170, 184, 185,
  188, 190
Vousden M 92
Voysey MHA 6

Wake R 61
Wal L 111, 112
Wallace H, Mulcahy L 137, 138

Walsh M, Ford P 71
ward sister x, xii, xiii, 2, 3, 4, 7, 8, 9, 11,
          70, 82, 83, 84, 92, 102, 111, 137,
          148, 152, 165, 186, 189
Warner M, Longley M, Gould E, Picek A
          82
Warnock M 40, 43
Warren J, Harris M 102
Waterlow J 111, 112
Watson H, Harris B 61
Watt N 116
Wellhouse NHS Trust 71
Wells-Pestell, Lord 14
Westminster Hospital 42
Wharrad HJ, Allcock N, Chapple M 68
While A 59, 64
While A, Roberts J, Fitzpatrick J 58, 59
White BJ 120
White E, Riley E, Davies S, Twinn S 59, 60
White M 41
Whittington Hospital 8
Wilderspin J 132

Wilkinson R 67
Willcock K 122
Williams C, Soothill K, Barry J 142, 145
Williams K 144, 145
Williams L 112
Williams M 70
Williams R, Fisher A 4, 9
Williams S, Michie S, Pattani S 116
Williamson J 110
Wilson-Barnett J 35, 101
Winson SKG 104
Winston, Lord 181
Winterton A 155, 174
Wise A 90
Wood CJ 5
Wright F W 20
Wright S 106, 107
Wright S, Gough P, Poulton B 105, 106
Wyatt JF 13

Yorston J 109
Young, Baroness 137